CHAPTER 1

Introduction and Literature Survey

Chapter One

Introduction and Literature Survey

1.1. The human prostate

The prostate gland is the largest accessory sex organ in males [1]. It is a fibromuscular and glandular structure lies just below the neck of the bladder and surrounds the urethra [2,3], anatomically, it has the shape of a compressed inverted cone [5]. The normal prostate in an adult weighs about 20 grams and contains the posterior urethra, which is about 2.5 centimeters in length [2]. It produces a thin, milky alkaline secretion that aids sperm motility by helping to maintain an optimum pH. The contraction of smooth muscle in the gland promotes semen expulsion during ejaculation [3].

The prostate is a complex organ consisting of acinar, stromal and muscular elements, structurally it is composed of fibromuscular tissue (30-50%) and glandular epithelial cells (50-70%) [4,5]. The glandular epithelium of the prostate consists of two layers: tall columnar luminal cells and flattened cuboidal basal cells. The epithelium rests on a thin basement membrane and the supporting stroma consists of equal amounts of smooth muscle and fibrous tissue [1].

There are three major regions within the normal prostate: the peripheral zone, the central zone and the periurethral transitional zone [4,6,7], as shown in Figure (1-1).

The peripheral and central zones which form a glandular portion are together constitute about 95% of the gland while the periurethral transitional zone constitute about only 5% of the gland [8]. Based on embryologic, ultrastructural and arterial injection studies, the prostate is now regarded as essentially two separate organs as shown in Figure (1-2),

1. The periurethral transitional, female portion, which is sensitive to androgens and estrogens, and this represents the inner group of glands, commonly referred to as the female prostate. It gives rise to benign nodular hyperplasia. For this reason benign enlargement mainly produces urinary symptoms.

2. Subcapsular true male prostate, which is sensitive to androgens; the latter forms a horseshoe-like sheath around the former [1].

Smooth muscle cells are found throughout the prostate, but in the upper part of the prostate and bladder neck (the internal sphincter) these subserve a sexual function, closing during ejaculation. Resection of this tissue during prostatectomy is responsible for retrograde ejaculation (dry ejaculation) [8].

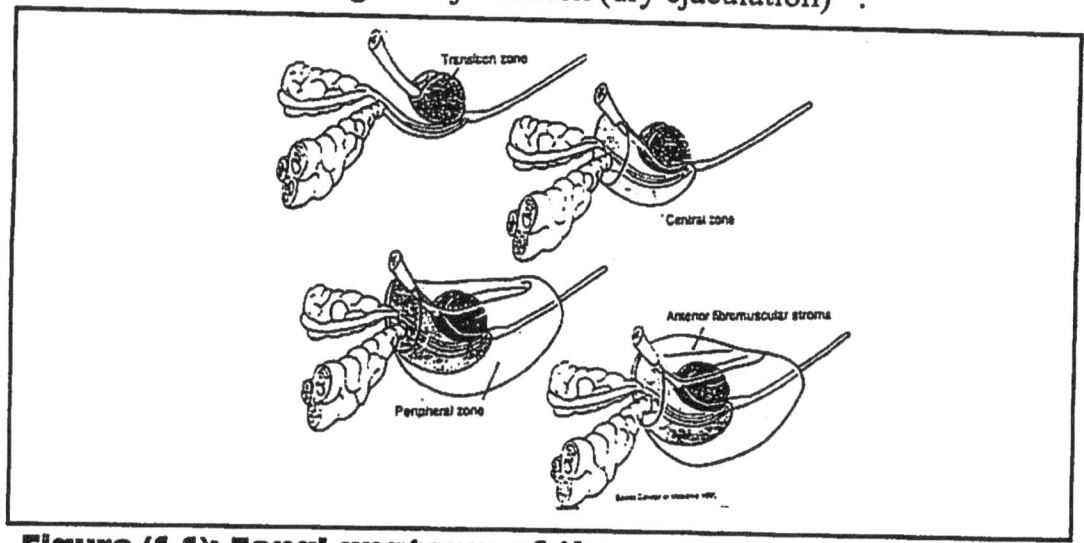

Figure (1-1): Zonal anatomy of the prostate: the three glandular zones of the prostate and the anterior fibromuscular stroma [6].

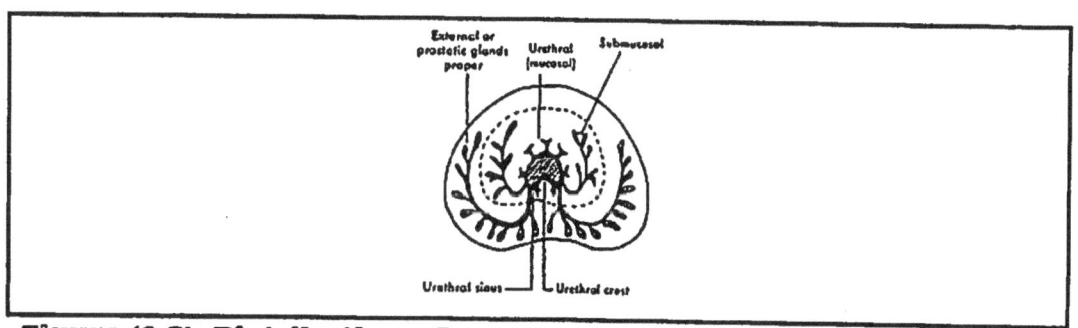

Figure (1-2): Distribution of normal prostatic glands slightly modified. Urethral (mucosal) and submucosal glands together form inner group, which is separated from outer gland group by an inconstant capsule [1]

1.2. Pathology of prostate [1]

The most common prostate pathological conditions may be classified according to following:

1. Non-tumorous conditions; these include:
   - Acute prostatitis
   - Chronic prostatitis
   - Granulomatous prostatitis

- Corpora amylacea and calculi
- Thrombosis and infarction

2. Tumorous conditions; these are subdivided into:

- **Tumorlike lesions:** such as prostatic cysts, amyloid deposits and prostatic hyperplasia.

- **Benign tumors:** such as adenomas, fibroadenomas, fibromas or leiomyomas.

- **Malignant tumors:** which includes various types of prostatic carcinoma.

1.2.1. Benign prostatic hyperplasia (BPH)

Incidence

Benign prostatic hyperplasia (BPH) is an age-related non-malignant enlargement of the prostate gland. It is one of the most common diseases of aging men [3]. It seldom occurs before the age of 50, but the incidence increases with age, and it can be found in 75% to 80% of men over age 80 [1].

Etiology

The exact cause of benign prostatic hyperplasia is unclear [3]. The fact that the condition occurs largely in older men suggests a relationship to changes in hormone balance associated with aging [3, 9-14].

Both androgens and estrogens appear to contribute to the process by having a synergistic effect in the development of BPH [9,12,14,15,16].

It has been postulated that the increase in levels of estrogen that occurs with aging may facilitate the synergistic action of androgens and estrogens despite a decline in testicular output of testosterone [3] on the ambisexual sensitive tissue of the periurethral prostatic area [1], produces irregular hyperplasia of the gland [17].

Finally, many investigators in their clinical reports have pointed to sexual indulgence or perversion as etiologic factors [1].

Symptoms

Because the prostate encircles the urethra, BPH exerts its effect through obstruction of urinary outflow from the bladder; therefore, the symptoms of BPH may include the following: urinary frequency, weak stream, dysuria and nocturia [3,15,18].

In the latter stages of BPH the urinary obstruction can give rise to urinary tract infection (e.g. cystitis) and kidney damage [1,3,19,4].

Diagnosis

The diagnosis of BPH is based on a typical history and observation of urinary retention [3].

The disease can be diagnosed by a rectal examination, a smooth rubbery enlargement of the prostate is usually detected also diagnostic ultrasound, either transabdominal or transrectal, offers the ability to evaluate the kidneys, ureters and bladder. Abdominal x-rays may be used to reveal the size of the prostate gland and give information about the possible kidneys damage [3,19].

Blood and urine analyses are used as adjuncts to determine BPH complications. Urinalysis is done to detect bacteria, white blood cells, or microscopic hematuria in the presence of infection and inflammation. Elevations in serum creatinine and blood urea nitrogen (BUN) suggest renal damage [3].

Treatment

The mechanism by which the prostate restricts bladder outflow is thought to be partly due to a mechanical component caused by the bulk of the prostatic mass and partly to a dynamic muscular component resulting from stimulation of adrenergic alpha-receptors in the prostatic fibromuscular stroma, capsule and bladder neck [5,20,21]. Therefore , there are several options of treatment, these include:

1) Surgical treatments

Surgical removal of benign enlarged prostate can be accomplished by several techniques [5]:

a. Transurethral resection prostatectomy (TURP)

Is the most common technique. The principles of (TURP) are to remove the obstructing adenomatous portion of the prostate via the urethra using a transurethral resectoscope [5,20].

b. Open prostatectomy [2,15,19,8,22]

Three different surgical procedures are used:

- Suprapubic (transvesical) prostatectomy
- Retropubic prostatectomy
- Perineal prostatectomy

c. Laser prostatectomy [3,5]

The use of laser technology in the ablation of prostatic tissue is one of the new thermotherapies which has rapidly become a widely used procedure, the advantages of laser prostatectomy over TURP include technical simplicity, lack of complications such as bleeding, retrograde ejaculation, impotence and incontinence.

d. Microwave treatment [8]

Is one of the most newer treatments causing tissue destruction. It aims at providing an external source of microwaves, which are then focused within the prostate gland by intraurethral route.

2) Pharmacological treatment

- ### α_1-Adrenergic receptor blockers

The rationale for using alpha blockers in the treatment of BPH was based on the observation that the contractile properties of prostate smooth muscle are primarily mediated by α_1-adrenergic receptors [5,23].

Three selective α_1-blockers have been used to relieve urinary obstruction and increase urine flow: prazosin, doxazosin and terazosin. Orthostatic hypotension, dizziness and asthenia can be the side effects of the α-adrenergic blocking drugs[3,23].

3) Hormonal manipulation

Androgen deprivation provides a mean of shrinking the prostate, thereby relieving obstruction and improving quality of life. This can be achieved by medical castration, using drugs with antiandrogenic activity[7,21,23,24,25].

The use of antiandrogen therapy (e.g., flutamide, nilutamide) may have some beneficial effect upon BPH, but the cost to the patient (impotence) is too high [2].

There are several options of the hormonal treatment:

a. LH-RH Analogues: Such as leuprolide acetate, goserelin acetate and buserelin acetate. These analogues may act by initially stimulating pituitary gonadotropin production and then inhibiting it [3,15].

b. Antiandrogens: These drugs may act by the blocking androgen action at the end-organ receptor such as flutamide, nilutamide and casodex [26,27].

c. **5α-Reductase inhibitors:** Such as finasteride (proscar), these drugs may act by inhibition the conversion of testosterone to its more potent metabolite dihydrotestosterone (DHT) [23,26,27].

d. **Aromatase inhibitors:** Such as testolactone, aromatase is the enzyme that converts androgens to estrogens in the peripheral tissue. Estrogens are believed to act synergistically with androgens in controlling prostate growth; therefore aromatase inhibitors should diminish and improve symptoms by inhibition the testosterone conversion [5,21,27,28].

1.2.2. Prostate cancer (PCA)

Incidence

Prostate cancer is the most common male cancer in the United States and is second to lung cancer as a cause of cancer-related deaths in men [1,3]. The incidence increases with age; over 80% of all prostate cancers are diagnosed in men over the age of 65 [3]. It varies markedly from country to country and varies among races, for example, the incidence is more frequent in Caucasians and Negroes, and rare in Mongoloid races and Japanese [3,22].

Therefore both genetical and environmental factors affecting the incidence of prostate cancer.

Carcinoma of the prostate usually originates in the peripheral zone of the gland, this location is distant from urethra, and the growth is therefore initially asymptomatic [8].

Etiology and risk factors

Although the precise etiology of prostate cancer (PCA) is unknown, testosterone accelerates the activity of carcinoma cells, whereas orchiectomy or estrogen therapy causes regression of tumor. These observations have led to the theory that androgens are in some way responsible for carcinoma of the prostate. But prolonged administration of androgens has not produced any tumors, and cancer of the prostate occurs at the time of life when the level of androgens is normally low.

The most prevalent hypothesis is that carcinoma of the prostate, which is a slow–growing tumor, may begin at the stage of life when androgen levels are high[1,3,16].

Recently, it was found that married men and men with children have an increased risk of prostate cancer [6]. Also the genetic and environmental factors may be considered as etiologic factors of prostate cancer [3,16].

Types of prostate cancer

Four categories of prostate cancer are recognized [1,22,29]:

1. **Latent carcinoma:** These tumors exist but do not become manifest, i.e. they produce no clinical evidence of disease. This type is found in autopsies of men dying of other causes.

2. **Incidental carcinoma:** In 6-20% of tissues removed surgically for clinically BPH, histologic examination shows carcinoma of the prostate.

3. **Occult carcinoma:** It is found in a number of patients who have no symptoms of prostatic carcinoma and show evidence of metastases on clinical examination.

4. **Clinical carcinoma:** This includes all cases in which rectal examination has aroused suspicion of carcinoma of the prostate and the diagnosis is confirmed by pathologic examination of the tissue removed from the prostate.

Signs and symptoms

The only sign of prostatic carcinoma may be an abnormal rectal examination. Therefore any irregular, firm, or hard nodule palpable on rectal examination should be biopsied [5].

There are no distinct symptoms of early carcinoma of the prostate, and when present, they are indistinguishable from those of BPH, these include: hesitancy, nocturia, incomplete bladder emptying, diminished urinary stream, dysuria, hematuria, blood in the ejaculate, perineal pain and sudden development of impotence. Late cancers usually manifest themselves through low back pain, fatigue, weight loss, anemia and shortness of breath, which indicate bone metastases [1,3,6,30].

Diagnosis

The standard technique to delineate the local extent of disease is digital rectal examination (DRE) followed by computed tomography (CT) or magnetic resonance imaging (MRI) to delineate lymph node involvement. In the last ten years, transrectal ultrasonography (TRUS) with biopsy has been introduced to assess both volume of cancer within the prostate as well as extracapsular extension of prostate cancer, this method can detect the cancer as small as 5 mm in diameter. Bone scintigraphy is still the preferred method to rule out metastatic involvement; acid phosphatase is being used less commonly, while cancer diagnosis has been aided greatly by the availability of PSA [3,5].

Staging

In 1992, the American Joint Committee on Cancer (AJCC) and the International Union Against Cancer (IUAC) adopted a new TNM classification system that has now replaced the older Whitemore–Jewett (ABCD) Scheme. Table (1-1) shows a comparison of these two systems.

Table (1-1): Comparison of the TNM staging system and Whitemore-Jewett staging system [3,6,8,31].

Whitemore-Jewett	TNM
A: Non palpable, asymptomatic and diagnosed after TURP.	T_1: Clinical inapparent tumor, not palpable or visible by imaging and the tumor is surrounded by palpably normal gland.
A_1: – < 5% resected specimen.	T_{1a}: Tumor incidental histologic finding in 5% or less of tissue resected.
A_2:– >5 % resected specimen.	T_{1b}: Tumor incidental histologic finding in more than 5% of tissue resected.
B: Palpable on digital examination and has a smooth nodule deforming contour.	T_2: Tumor confined within prostate.
B_1: One lobe.	T_{2a}: Tumor involves half of a lobe or less. T_{2b}: Tumor involves more than half of a lobe, but not both lobes.
B_2: Both lobes.	T_{2c}: Tumor involves both lobes.
C: Capsular penetration but has not produced clinically evident metastasis.	T_3: Tumor extends through the prostatic capsule. T_{3a}: Unilateral extracapsular extension. T_{3b}: Bilateral extracapsular extension.
D: Extracapsular penetration	T_{3c}: Tumor invades seminal vesicle. T_4: Tumor invades adjacent structures other than seminal vesicles. T_{4a}: Tumor invades any of bladder neck, external sphincter, and rectum. T_{4b}: Tumor invades levator muscles and/or is fixed to pelvic wall.
D_1: Regional nodes	N: Regional lymph nodes.

D_2: Beyond regional nodes with distant metastasis	M: M/a Non regional nodes
	     M/b Bones
	     M/c Other sites

T: Primary tumor; N: Regional lymph nodes; M: Distant metastasis	

Treatment

There are several types of prostate cancer treatment:-

1. Radical prostatectomy

In the early stages the radical prostatectomy can be curative. It is indicated only if the tumor is confined to prostate gland and no metastasis detected [15].

Radical prostatectomy entails removal of the seminal vesicles and the prostate with its capsule. Modification in the surgical technique has led to improved continence and potency rates [32].

2. Radiation treatment

The indication for curative radiation treatment is given if the tumor is confined to the prostate and no metastatic spread is found, while palliative radiation is used in advanced stages [15].

3. Hormonal manipulation

Since the proliferation of prostatic cells is androgen–dependent, androgen ablation therapy is currently the first line of treatment for inoperable prostatic cancer [33]. This can be achieved by interfering with the hypothalamus–pituitary axis (extra prostatic) or by blocking the hormonal effect in the prostate (intra prostatic) [15].

(a) Bilateral orchiectomy

The basic treatment for advanced prostate cancer is the bilateral orchiectomy and is the most effective form of androgen ablation for androgens of testicular origin [5,15].

(b) Estrogen treatment

The estrogen administration suppresses pituitary LH–RH secretion, thereby reducing circulating testosterone to castrate levels. Diethylstilbestrol (DES) is the most commonly administered form of estrogen [34].

Recently it was known that the most important beneficial effect of estrogen treatment is by having a bone masspreserving capacity in elderly males with metastatic prostate cancer [35]. Gynecomastia, loss of libido and potency, voice changes, cardiovascular complications, fluid retention and vomiting are the chief side effects of estrogen therapy [6,3,34].

(c) LH-RH Analogues (Medical castration)

These drugs cause a down–regulation of the gonadotrophin receptors in the anterior lobe of the pituitary if given in supraphysiological doses over a prolonged time. After initial stimulation of the gonadotrophin release is inhibited and the peripheral testosterone level falls to castrate range within two weeks [3,15,20,36].

(d) Antiandrogens

Antiandrogens may act by inhibition of androgen synthesis or inhibition of androgen action [5].

Inhibitors of androgen synthesis include aminoglutethimide, ketoconazole and spironolactone. Ketoconazole is a synthetic imidazole analog initially used as antifungal agent. The mechanism of action involves inhibition of cytochrome P450–dependent enzymes; therefore both adrenal and testicular androgen synthesis are inhibited [5,32]. Antiandrogens that act by competing with testosterone and dihydrotestosterone for binding to the prostatic androgen receptors can be divided into two groups: **The steroidal antiandrogens,** e.g., cyproterone acetate, megestrol acetate and **the nonsteroidal antiandrogens,** e.g., flutamide, nilutamide and bicalutamide (Casodex).

The steroidal antiandrogens block androgen action, but have in addition progestational and glucocorticoid activities and are, therefore , called non–selective antiandrogens [37]. Their progestational activity results in a downregulation of luteinizing hormone–releasing hormone, and consequently of luteinizing hormone, testosterone, and 5α-DHT. The nonsteroidal antiandrogens also block androgen action, however, they stimulate the hypothalamus–pituitary–gonadal axis, and consequently lead to increased testosterone and DHT levels, and are therefore also referred to as selective antiandrogens [32,37].

(e) Combined androgen blockade (CAB)

Following medical or surgical castration, serum testosterone concentrations are reduced by approximately 95%, but androgens of adrenal origin are not suppressed [37]. The concept of CAB is that of abolishing the testicular secretion of testosterone by means of orchidectomy or the use of LH–RH therapy and then inhibiting the effects of adrenal androgenic steroids by means of androgen receptor blockade [8]. Combined use of an LH–RH analogue and flutamide has provided better results, particularly in men with minimal disease [3].

4. Cytotoxic chemotherapy

Due to the severe side effects of chemotherapy in older patients, this treatment should only be considered if all other modalities have failed.

Chemotherapeutic agents such as estramustin phosphate, 5-fluorouracil, cyclophosphamide and cisplatin have been tested with some success [2,15].

The choice of patient treatment type depends primarily on the stage of the disease, therefore , men with stage A_1 are usually treated with watchful waiting unless they are relatively young. Radical prostatectomy and radiation therapy are used as curative methods of treatment in early disease that is limited to the prostate (stages A_2 and B). The use of nerve–sparing methods of radical prostatectomy has improved the outcomes of surgical intervention. Radiation therapy is being used increasingly in the treatment of (stage C) disease. Metastatic disease (stage D) is usually treated with antiandrogen therapy. Orchiectomy or estrogen therapy is often effective in reducing symptoms and extending survival [3].

1.3. Tumor markers

Tumor markers are substances that are produced by tumor cells or substances released from normal cells in response to the presence of tumor; therefore disappearance of the marker should indicate eradication of the tumor, whereas an increase in marker concentration should indicate tumor growth [3,46,47].

Some substances such as hormones and enzymes are produced normally by the tissue involved but become overexpressed as a result of cancer. Other tumor markers, such as oncofetal proteins, are produced during fetal development and are induced to reappear later in life as a result of benign and malignant neoplasms [3].

Many tumor markers that are produced by the tumor cells, their levels would be dependent on the mass of the tumor, and may be influenced by a variety of factors, among them, the number of tumor cells, the proportion of tumor cells synthesizing the marker, the synthetic rate per cell, the location of tumor marker within the cell and the mechanism of release from the cell, therefore, the quantity of tumor marker should indicate how much tumor was present (tumor burden) and to what stage the tumor has progressed [48,49].

Few markers are specific for a single individual tumor (tumor–specific markers); most are found with different tumors of the same tissue type (tumors– associated markers) [46]. Table (1-2) lists useful tumor markers in screening, in determining therapy, in providing prognostic information, in monitoring the response to therapy and in detecting relapse, also they are useful in early detection of local recurrence of malignant disease after treatment, or in detecting the development of metastasis [3,50].

Circulated tumor markers can be measured chemically, immunologically (i.e. radioimmuno assay, immunoradiometric assay, immunofluorescence assay) and molecular biologically [46].

Table (1-2): Tumor markers, classified according to biochemical and biological characteristics, and their associated malignancies (46,49,50-53).

Marker type	Example	Associated malignancies
Oncofetal antigens	Carcinoembryonic antigen (CEA)	Colorectal, breast, lung and pancrease
	Alpha-fetoprotein (AFP)	Germ cell tumors & hepatoma
Cancer associated antigens (Glycoproteins)	CA 15-3	Breast
	CA 19-9	Pancreatic & gastrointestinal
	CA 125	Ovarian
	Prostate specific antigen (PSA)	Prostate
Hormones	Parathyroid hormone (PTH)	Hepatoma, renal cell & parathyroid
	Antidiuretic hormone (ADH)	Small cell lung cancer
	Human calcitonine (hCT)	Medullary thyroid cancer
	Beta core human chorionic gonadotropin (β-core-hCG)	Cervical, ovarian, testicular and endometrial cancers
Enzymes	Neuron specific enolase (NSE)	Neuroblastoma, thyroid medullary carcinoma & small-cell lung cancer
	Cathepsin D (Cath-D)	Breast
	Prostatic acid phosphatase (PAP)	Prostate
	Terminal deoxynucleotidyl transferase (TdT)	Acute lymphoblastic leukemia
	Lactate dehydrogenase (LDH)	Most malignancies
Proteins	Thyroglobulin	Thyroid
	Ferritin	Pancreatic & breast
	Immunoglobulins	Lymphoma & myeloma
	Beta 2-microglobulin (β2-M)	Multiple myeloma
Receptor-site proteins	Epidermal growth factor receptor (EGF-R)	Breast, bladder, renal, head and neck
	Estrogen and progesterone receptors (ER & PR)	Breast & uterine
Neuromediators	Catechol amine metabolites (24-hour urine)	Neuroblastoma
	5-hydroxyindol acetic acid (24-hours urine)	Carcinoid
Oncogenes	c-erb B-2 (or HER-2/neu)	Breast & stomach
	myc c-myc	Colon cancer
	N-myc	Neuroblastoma
Virus	Human papilloma virus (HPV)	Genital cancers (cervical, vulval & penile)
Cytogenetic markers	P53 gene	Colorectal
	Philadelphia chromosome (Ph¹)	Chronic myeloid leukemia

1.4. Tumor markers of prostate cancer

The important tumor markers of prostate cancer are:

Prostate specific antigen (PSA)

PSA is a 34–kDa glycoprotein with a serine protease activity, secreted into the cytoplasm of normal, benign and malignant prostatic cells and is found in no other normal tissues or tumors [3,55].

Normally the function of PSA is in aiding liquefaction of semen. It was considered the product of the human glandular Kallikrein gene locus on chromosome 19 and is almost exclusively expressed in the prostate [31].

Serum PSA (S.PSA) content is increased in benign prostatic disease (prostatitis, BPH), as well as in cancer. However, there is a clear relationship between plasma PSA content and stage of PCA [6]. S.PSA has to date been recognized as the most useful marker for early diagnosis, staging of locally confined disease, and can give an indication of the presence of lymph node metastases, also during watchful waiting regimen or during androgen deprivation therapy (ADT), S.PSA is the most reliable marker for surveillance, for example, the treatment of BPH and PCA with ADT usually decrease the S.PSA concentration. Hence, S.PSA is a valuable tumor marker for prognosticating the response to ADT, and so detectable levels of S.PSA after radical prostatectomy option suggest persistent local of metastatic disease [3,31,46,57,58].

Prostatic acid phosphatase (PAP)

Acid phosphatase (ACP) [E.C. 3.1.3.2] is the name given a group of phosphohydrolases that hydrolyze phosphoric monoesters at an acidic pH and is the first marker found to be associated with a human cancer [6]. Several ACP isoenzymes are found in human tissues and cells including liver, spleen, kidney, prostate, erythrocytes, platelets, osteoclasts and hairy cell leukemia [6,53].

The prostatic acid phosphatase(PAP) is produced in normal prostatic tissue as well as malignant prostatic tissue which is completely inhibited by L–tartarate (tartarate–labile–isoenzyme) [3].

Patients with prostatic carcinoma that has metastasized have elevated serum levels of total ACP and PAP, while patients with prostate cancer (PCA) still confined within the capsule and also patients with (BPH) usually have normal levels of this enzyme.

Thus, ACP or PAP determination is useful in diagnosing metastatic PCA but is of little value in diagnosing the early stages of this disease and therefore PSA was considered a more reliable marker than PAP and so PSA has largely replaced ACP and PAP in evaluating patients with PCA [6,53-56].

PSA-density (PSAD)

Since PSA is produced by the normal prostate and BPH, serum levels can be compared with the volume of the prostate gland or the transition zone (BPH adenomas). The ratio of PSA to gland volume is the PSA density, measured in nanograms per milliliter per cubic centimeter of prostate tissue. Since PSA released into the serum is greater per gram of cancer tissue than per gram of BPH tissue, the PSAD should help to discriminate cancer from BPH. However, PSAD is still being evaluated as a prognostic factor and the value of this test remains controversia l[6].

DNA ploidy

DNA ploidy has recently been reported to be useful in predicting prognosis in PCA. Several studies have shown that low–grade tumors are associated with diploidy and high–grade tumors with aneuploidy.

Studies by Tribukait have also suggested that patients with diploid tumors do well with expectant therapy while those with aneuploidy do poorly [5,6,31,59,60].

CA 195 & CA 549

These tumor markers have been reported to be elevated in sera of patients with PCA in addition to another types of malignancies, they are approved only for investigational use in the United States [49].

Serum TPS (Tissue polypeptide-specific antigen)

Serum TPS has been observed to be characteristic of PCA proliferation, and increased levels of TPS seem to be closely related to tumor progression. Serial measurement of this marker could be useful in the early diagnosis of a relapse after radical prostatectomy [61].

CK-BB

The BB isozyme of creatine kinase has been found in significant concentration in the serum and pleural fluid of patients with PCA. If the ratio of CK1 (BB-isozyme) in pleural effusion fluid to that in serum is greater than 3.7, the probability is high that a malignant tumor is the cause. The ratio of patients with a benign course of pleural effusions was less than 1.6 [50,55,62].

Molecular markers

The molecular markers under investigation include oncogenes and tumor suppressor genes. For example, $nm23-H_2$ mRNA levels have been shown to correlate with higher stage cancers [64] and levels of $nm23-H_1$ and $nm23-H_2$ expression were reduced in metastasis relative to primary tumors. Similarly, the P53 (a tumor suppressor gene, clearly plays a role in many cancers but its role in PCA remains controversial) mutations occur in only a small proportion of early stage PCA, but in a higher proportion of metastatic lesions [6,63].

These data suggest that further delineation of the role of these newer markers will lead to a much better understanding of the pathways of PCA progression and to improved prognostic indices [6].

1.5. Hormones and prostate

The understanding of the hormonal regulation of normal and diseased human prostates is incomplete [38], but it was known that the prostate cancer differs in various endocrinological aspects from the BPH and also from the normal human prostate [39].

The main hormones acting on the prostate are:

1. Androgens

Androgens play an important role in male physiology and pathology [25]. The prostate gland is completely dependent upon androgens both for normal growth and functions and also for abnormal growth, since neither cancer nor hyperplasia develops in castrates [38].

Therefore , it can be considered that androgens are the principal hormonal regulators for normal and abnormal growth [40], and the degree of androgen sensitivity determines the patients initial response to androgen deprivation therapies [5].

2. Estrogens

The presence of estrogen receptors in human prostatic tissue is largely confined to a periurethral stromal cells [28].

Some evidence has accrued to suggest that the amount of androgen receptor in the human prostate may be increased by treatment with estrogens, thus increased estrogen levels with age in men could accelerate prostatic growth in the face of a declining or static androgen production [14].

3. Prolactin

The prolactin stimulates proliferation of normal, hyperplastic and malignant human cells in culture [41,42]. It is generally accepted that the growth promoting actions of prolactin involve interaction of the hormone with its receptor in the plasma membrane of prostatic cell [43], this interaction increases the uptake of testosterone whereas estrogens inhibit this binding and thereby inhibit the uptake of testosterone by the prostate cells [13,44]. Another investigators showed that there was a synergistic relationship between prolactin and testosterone, also the mechanism by which prolactin affects the androgenic response is not clear but probably prolactin may affect the androgen binding protein/receptor level of the prostate gland [45].

The potential pathways of hormonal influences on prostate cancer with different hormonal treatment routes are depicated in Figure (1-3).

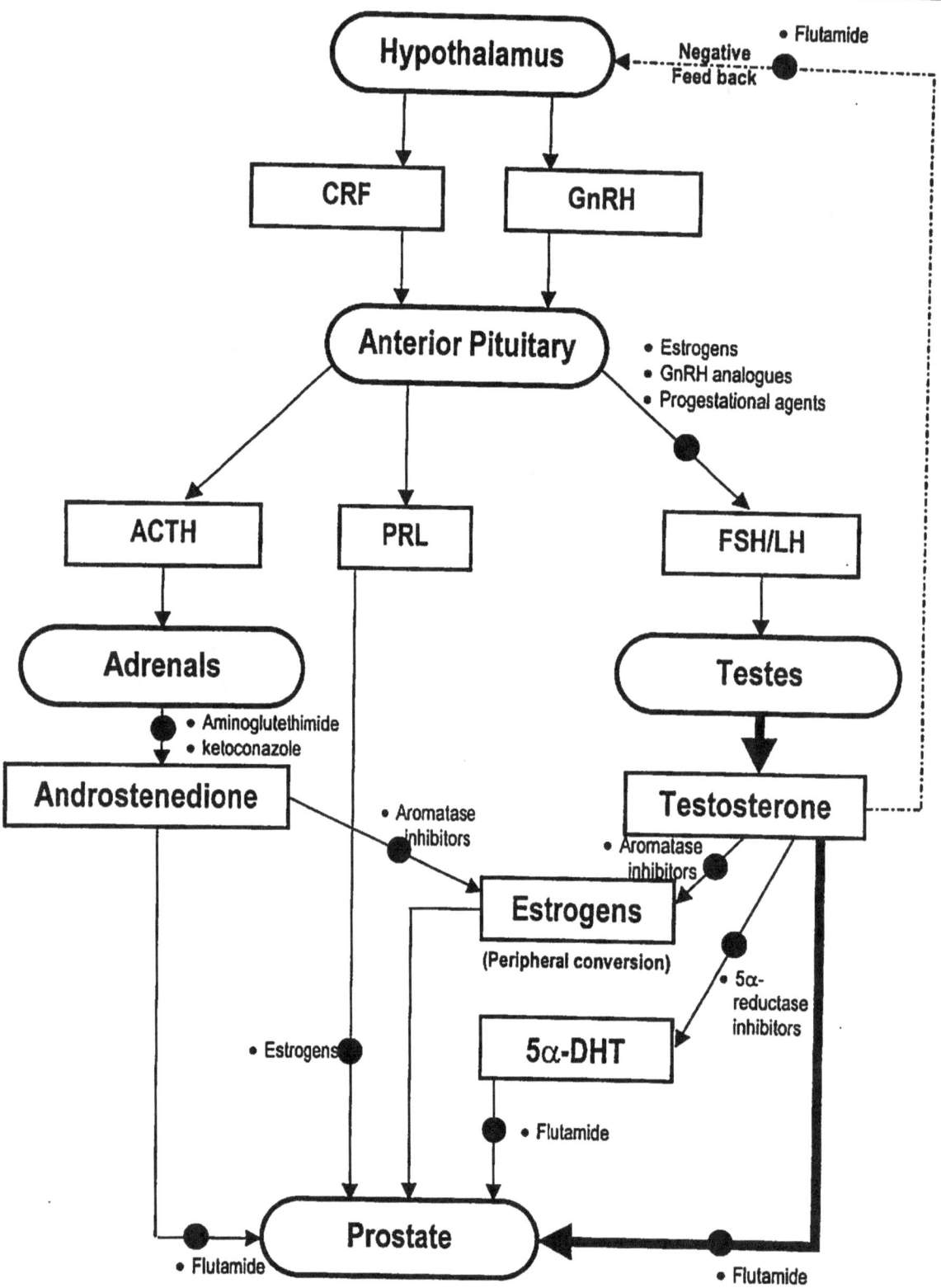

Figure (1-3): Endocrine relationships among adrenal glands, testes, pituitary, and hypothalamus. Point of inhibition and the drugs of treatment of prostate cancer that are active at that site are indicated. CRF, corticotropin releasing factor; GnRH, gonadotropin releasing hormone; FSH, follicle stimulating hormone; LH, luteinizing hormone, ACTH, corticotropin; PRL, prolactin [5,6].

1.6. Steroid hormones

Steroids are a group of lipids based on a skeleton of four fused rings (the perhydrocyclopentanephenanthrene system). They are classified depending on the number of carbon atoms of the molecules into: **progesterones, glucocorticoids and minerlcorticoids** with 21, androgens with 19 and estrogens with 18 carbon atoms. Steroid hormones are synthesized through a series of enzymatic reactions starting with a common precursor, cholesterol, which serves as the basic for all steroid hormones [65,66].

They are water-insoluble compounds that are transported in the blood stream to their site of action by binding to proteins in the plasma; therefore it is generally believed that only the free steroid can enter cells and the steroids can freely diffuse across the plasma membranes of all cells but are sequestered only within cells that contain specific intracellular receptors [53,67,68].

Steroid hormones exert long–term effects (hours or even days) on their target cells; they stimulate cell growth and differentiation and regulate the synthesis of specific proteins primarily by altering the rate of transcription of specific genes. Steroids exert these actions on target cells after binding to specific receptors, which are localized primarily within the nucleus [66-69,71].

The steroid hormones are converted by the liver to inactive compounds by a group of hepatic catabolic enzymes such as hydrogenases, dehydrogenases and hydroxylases [53].

Androgens are a group of C19 steroids that secreted mainly by the testes and, to a lesser degree, by the adrenal cortex and ovary. In males, they are involved in the development and maintenance of secondary sexual characteristics and several physiological functions, such as normal reproduction, sex drive, sexual performance, skeleton and skeletal muscle growth and development during puberty. In females, they stimulate growth of pubic hair and probably libido, besides acting as estrogen precursors [46,55,72,73].

1.7. Testosterone

The most potent androgen is testosterone (T). It is secreted mainly by the leydig cells of the testis. The secretion is under the regulation of pituitary gland via a trophic hormone, luteinizing hormone (LH) [26].

Adrenal cortex and ovary secrete very little testosterone. Normally they secrete less potent androgens, such as androstenedione, dehydroepiandrosterone (DHA) and dehydroepiandrosterone sulfate (DHAS), which are metabolized to testosterone in most peripheral tissues [72,74].

Testosterone is converted to its metabolite, 5α-DHT by the 5α-reductase, an NADPH-dependent enzyme, this conversion dose not occur in all androgen target tissues and it depends primarily on the type of tissue and the presence or absence of the 5α-reductase activity [70,74–76,97]. For example, prostate, seminal vesicles and skin depend largely on 5α-DHT [77,78,98] while in kidney, skeletal muscle, female uterus and testes, testosterone may be the active form [79-82].

During puberty testosterone with or without DHT causes enlargement of the penis, seminal vesicles, muscle mass, larynex and thickening of the vocal cords, resulting in a deeper voice. Although testosterone is the major local hormone required for initiation and maintenance of spermatogenesis, DHT may participate in sperm production as well [70].

In subsequent adult life administration of testosterone causes nitrogen retention in both sexes, reflecting protein anabolism, therefore many athletes use testosterone and its derivatives to develop muscle and increase strength [70,72,83]. Testosterone has important effects on lipid metabolism, it increases circulating VLDL and LDL cholesterol while decreases circulating HDL cholesterol and favors accumulation of upper body, abdominal, and visceral fat. These lipid abnormalities are associated with an increased risk of cardiovascular disease [70].

Certain other diverse androgenic action can be ascribed to testosterone, these include [49,70,75,83-86,95]:

1) Initiation of sexual drive (libido) and the ability to achieve a physiologically complete erection (potency).

2) Suppression of mammary gland growth.

3) Stimulation of hematopoiesis and maintenance of a normal red blood cell mass.

4) Development of secondary sex organs, the prostate and seminal vesicles.

5) Stimulation of renal sodium reabsorption.

6) Suppression of hepatic synthesis of sex steroid–binding globulin (SSBG), corticosteroid–binding globulin (CBG) and thyroxine–binding globulin (TBG).

In boys and men testosterone measurement is related to the investigation of testicular dysfunction. Increased testosterone levels can be found in complete androgen resistance (testicular feminization). Common causes of decreased testosterone levels in males include: **hypogonadism, orchidectomy, estrogen** therapy, **Klinefelter's syndrome, hypopituitarism** and **hepatic cirrhosis.** Testosterone measurement has also been used to monitor the treatment by antiandrogen therapy for patients with PCA [84].

In women, it is useful in evaluating **hirsutism, alopecia** and **menstrual disorders,** common causes of increased serum testosterone levels include polycystic ovaries **(Stein-Leventhal syndrome),** ovarian and adrenal tumors[84,87,88].

Mechanism of testosterone action

The complex mechanism of androgen action at the cellular level has recently been clarified. Testosterone diffuses freely into cells, in many but not all target cells it rapidly undergoes reduction to 5α–DHT. However, testosterone and 5α–DHT are capable of binding to a single cytoplasmic receptor but with different affinities [5,53,70].

The native cytoplasmic receptors exist in inactive form, possibly in association with blocking proteins (Heat shock proteins). Binding of the testosterone to the C–terminus domain activates the cytoplasmic receptor by causing its dissociation from heat shock protein (transformation) and subsequent translocation into the target cell nucleus [6,70].

The activated testosterone–receptor complex dimerizes and the DNA–binding fingers of the receptor interact with a hormone response element (HRE) on a target DNA molecule. HREs are generally 8 to 15 base pairs long. Occupancy of the HRE activates various promotor elements on the DNA molecule. The testosterone–activated promotor nucleotide sequences initiate transcription at the start site of the specific gene message by RNA polymerase II. The resultant "immature" RNA then undergoes maturation to messenger RNA by capping, excision of untranslated nucleotide sequences, and splicing. Translation of the RNA message in the cytoplasm results in synthesis of specific target proteins (enzymes, structural proteins, receptor proteins, transcriptional proteins that will regulate the expression of other genes and proteins that are exported by the cell)[5,53,67,70].

Structure of the human androgen receptor (hAR)

The androgen receptor (AR) is a member of the superfamily of ligand activated nuclear transcription factors. It mediates the action of androgens at the level of transcriptional regulation. HAR has a calculated molecular weight of ~98000 Da and is composed of ~900–920 amino acids, the number varying owing the polymorphism in the length of poly glutamine and poly glycine tracts found in the N–terminal region of the receptor [33,74].

ARs, like other members of the nuclear receptor family, are composed of three functional domains [74,75,89,90]:

1. N-terminal domain

It contains 555 amino acids and makes up more than half of the AR protein. A striking feature of this domain is the presence of multiple amino acids repeats. In particular, repeats of poly glutamine (16–39 residues) and poly glycine (3–18 residues) are present in hAR as shown in Figure (1-4).

Epidemiological studies have shown that individuals with shorter repeats have a greater risk of developing prostate cancer [74].

It has been proposed that increased AR–transcriptional activity, with shorter glutamine repeat lengths, might be responsible for this increased risk of PCA, as AR–transcrptional activity is inversely related to the glutamine repeat length [74].

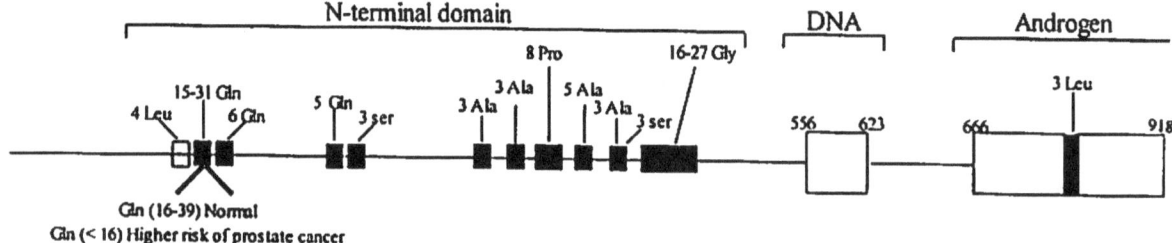

Figure (1-4): Schematic diagram of the domain structure of the hAR, the positions of oligo– and poly amino acid tracts are indicated [74,75].

2. DNA–binding domain

It consists of about 70 amino acids and is located between the N-terminal domain and the C-terminal ligand–binding domain. The amino acid sequence of this domain is similar among different steroid receptors (56–79% identity) and is identical in ARs from a variety of mammals. The DNA–binding domain contains two Zn^{2+} ions coordinated to the sulfurs of eight cysteins, which produces a helix–loop–helix structural domain that interacts with specific DNA sequences, termed androgen response elements (AREs) [74], as shown in Figure (1-5).

3. Hinge domain

This domain has about 30 amino acids that are located between the DNA–binding domain and the androgen–binding domain in the carboxyl–terminus of the AR. A nuclear localization (n_L, Figure (1-5)) signal that functions indepently of the DNA–binding domain is present in this domain. A related amino acid sequence has been shown to be important in nuclear localization of other steroid receptors and some other nuclear proteins [75].

4. Androgen–binding domain

The C–terminal androgen–binding domain contains about 290 amino acids and represents about 30% of the receptor. The ligand–binding domains of ARs from humans, rats and mice are identical, and sequence homology with other steroid receptors ranges between 15% and 54%. In addition to binding androgen, the ligand–binding domain also participates in transcriptional activation and receptor dimerization. ARs, as well as other steroid receptors, also interact with heat shock proteins through their ligand–binding domains in the inactivated states[33,74,91].

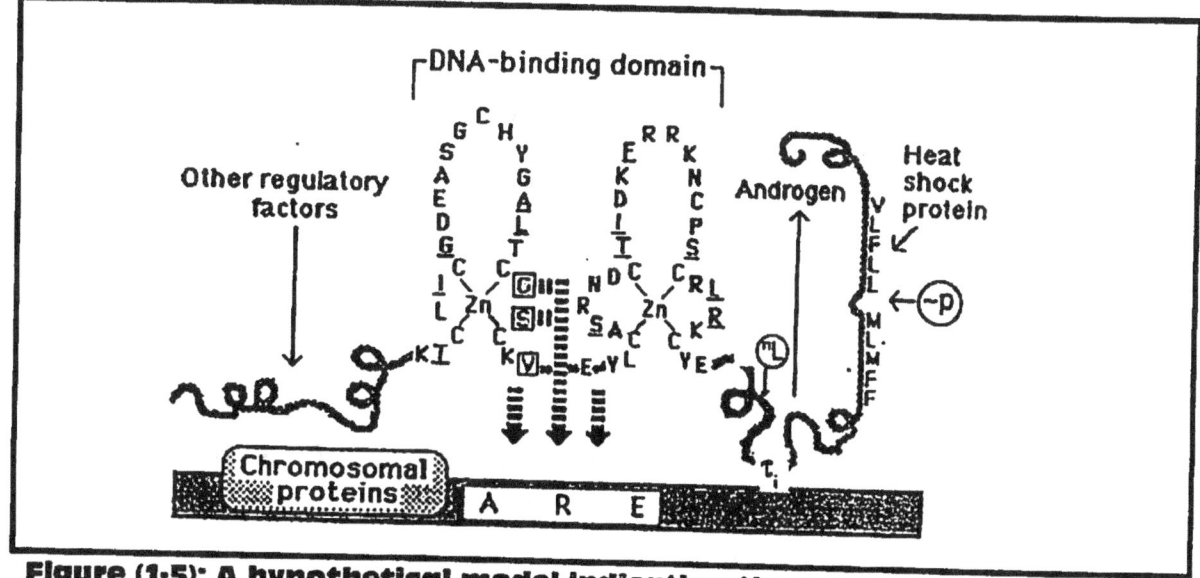

Figure (1-5): A hypothetical model indicating the roles of AR domains [75].

The gene encoding the hAR is located on the X-chromosome and has a size of > 90 Kb, it consists of eight exons, the first encoding the large N-terminal domain, the second and third encoding one Zinc finger element each, and the fourth through eighth exons encoding the androgen–binding domain [33,37], as shown in Figure (1–6).

1.8. Human androgen receptor (HAR) and prostate cancer (PCA)

Prostate cancer, like the gland from which it arises, is initially androgen dependent; therefore the front line therapy for metastatic prostate cancer (PCA) has been based on methods designed to prevent androgenic stimulation of the tumor. However, many of these tumors, while initially responding to androgen ablation therapy, eventually reoccur. The mechanism for this loss of dependence on androgens is not clear. Metastatic tumors often express AR, so loss of AR is not the reason for lack of androgenic growth control. AR is mutated in some prostate cancer cells, and in some cases these mutations change the properties of AR, such as ligand–binding specificity, which might allow AR to function in the absence of its normal ligand or in the presence of antiandrogen that function as agonists, not antagonists [74,99,100].

Also, it was shown that there is an amplification of the AR gene occurred during hormonal therapy and the levels of AR mRNA increased in patients showing gene amplification. Thus, it seems that AR gene amplification is one of the mechanisms by which tumor cells adapt to an environment with low androgen supply, and therefore failure of conventional androgen deprivation therapies of PCA [29,92,96,98].

Several somatic mutations have been detected in tumor specimens of patients with PCA. Most of the reported mutations are localized in the androgen–binding domain. A relatively high frequency of the Thr^{868} Ala mutation is particularly found in metastatic lesions (bone metastases) of PCA and can be considered as a hot spot as shown in Figure (1-7).

It was concluded that threonine on position 868 of the hAR limits the ligand specificity of the receptor to androgens [33,37,94].

It has been also shown that shorter CAG repeats of hAR gene are associated with a higher risk of PCA [93].

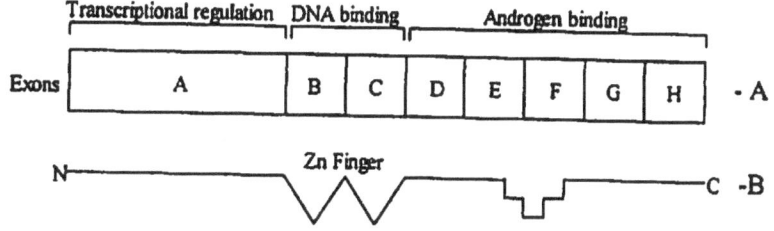

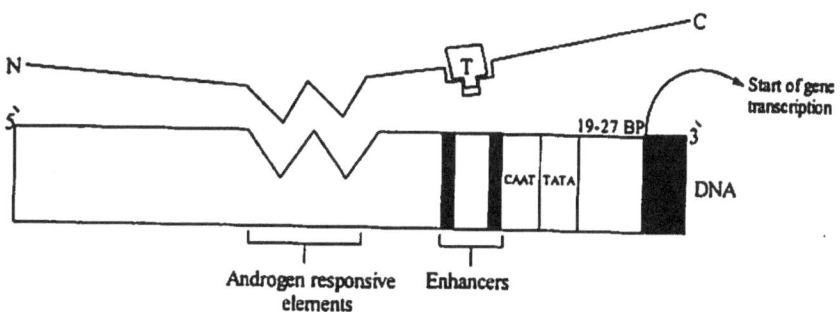

Figure (1-6): A: Diagrammatic representation of the AR gene divided into its 8 exons.
B: the organization of androgen–responsive gene. Testosterone binding activates the receptor, and it binds to the androgen response elements of the gene (as a dimer; not shown). Enhancers as well as a CAAT and a TATA box are present. Gene transcription begins 19-27 base pairs downstream of the TATA box[5].

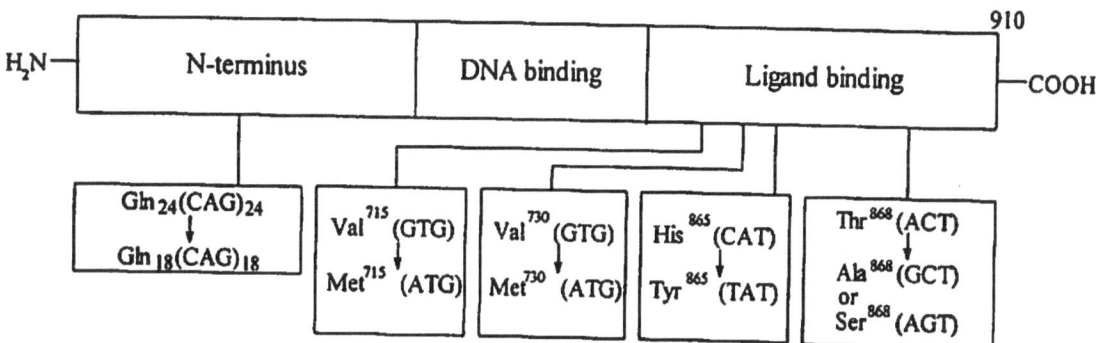

Figure (1-7): AR mutations detected in prostatic carcinoma tissue and in tumor cell line LNCaP [33,37].

Aim of the Work

The aim of the work in this thesis includes the following:

1. Determination of some biochemical constituents (testosterone, iron, copper, zinc, calcium and magnesium) in sera of normal men and patients with some tumors of prostate.

2. Measurement of testosterone levels in tissues of some prostatic tumors.

3. Development of a radioreceptor assay for testosterone receptors measurement in some tumors of prostate.

4. Molecular characterization of the binding of ^{125}I-testosterone with its crude prostatic tumors receptors and then studying the effect of various factors on these binding reactions (temperature, time, pH, testosterone concentration, receptor concentration, different salts and halides).

5. Developing a method for purification and isolation of testosterone receptors in human prostatic tumors.

6. Molecular characterization of the binding of ^{125}I-testosterone with its purified prostatic tumors receptors and studying the effect of various factors on these binding reactions (temperature, time, pH, testosterone concentration, and receptor concentration).

7. Determination of the kinetic and thermodynamic parameters of the binding reactions of testosterone with its receptors in human prostatic tumors.

8. Spectroscopic studies on the purified testosterone receptors in human prostatic tumors.

CHAPTER 2

Experimental Work

Experimental Work

2.1. Chemicals, Instruments and Tissue specimens used

2.1.1. Chemicals

All common laboratory chemicals and reagents were of analar grade and were used without further purification. Tris[hydroxymethyl] amino-methane, $MgCl_2$, $MnCl_2$, NaCl, Charcoal, Bovine serum albumin, Citric acid, Calf thymus DNA and Gelatin were obtained from Fluka.

EDTA (disodium salt), Na, K-tartarate, $CuSO_4.5H_2O$, NaF, Glycerol and β-mercaptoethanol were obtained from BDH.

Sephadex G-200, Dextran T-70, Blue dextran 2000 were obtained from Pharmacia Fine Chemicals, Switzerland.

Kit of radioactive testosterone (^{125}I-testosterone) was purchased from DiaSorin Corporation (USA). The activity of labeled testosterone was approximately 4 μci.

2.1.2. Instruments

The instruments used in this work were, LKB gamma counter type 1270 Rack gamma II, cooling centrifuge type Hettich, LKB spectrophotometer Ultraspec type 4050, sonicator (MSE soniprep 150), Shimadzu U.V-Visible recorder spectrophotometer type U.V.-160, Pye-Unicam pH meter, Memmert water bath, SM-Shaker, Memmert incubator and Perkin-Elmer type 5000 Atomic absorption spectrophotometer.

2.1.3. Patients

Two groups of prostatic tumors patients were included in this study. Group I contained 25 patients with (BPH). Group II consisted of 3 patients with (PCA). All tumors are without any type of prostatitis and patients were admitted for transurethral resection prostatectomy (TURP) treatment to the Saddam College of Medicine–University Hospital, Al-Mustansiriya Private Hospital and Al-Saddoon Private Hospital. They were histologically proven through the supervision of specialists at the Saddam College of Medicine–University Hospital and Al-Saddoon Private Hospital. The patients were newly diagnosed and not underwent of any type of therapy. Patients suffered from any disease that may interfere with our study were excluded. The host information of all patients and normal healthy subjects is summarized in Table (2-1).

Table (2-1): The host information of prostatic tumors patients and healthy subjects studied.

Groups	Number	Age (year)	Type of tumors
Benign	25	65.96±1.15	B.P.H
Malignant	3	73.66±0.62	2 patients with PCA stage D (metastasis)
			1 patient with PCA stage B (intracapsular)
Control	16	68±1.9	Age matched healthy individuals

2.1.4. Preparation of blood samples

Five milliliters of blood samples were obtained from patients undergoing TURP by venipuncture just before surgery. Sixteen physically normal age matched volunteers were used as controls. Blood samples were left for 20 min at room temperature. After coagulation, sera were separated by centrifugation at 2000 xg for 10 min, then sera were aspirated and stored in caped sterilized tubes at -20°C until time of analysis.

2.1.5. Collection of specimens

Human prostate tumors were obtained by transurethral resection prostatectomy (TURP). Fresh prostatic chips were immediately immersed in ice-cold isotonic saline solution. They were collected individually in plastic receptacle and stored at - 20°C until homogenization.

2.1.6. Preparation of prostatic tumors tissues homogenates

The frozen tissues were weighed, sliced finely with a scalpel in Petri dish standing on ice bath, the slices were thawed and further minced with scissors then homogenized in TEMG buffer with a ratio of 1:5 (weight: volume) using a manual homogenizer. The homogenate was filtered through four layers of nylon gauze in order to eliminate fibers of connective tissues, then centrifuged at 2000 xg for 75 min at 4°C. The sediment was suspended in 10 volumes of the TEMG buffer for 15 min at 4°C and then the suspension was used to obtain the crude nuclear fraction and the supernatant was used as crude cytosolic fraction [65].

2.1.7. Buffers and reagents

All buffer solutions were prepared [101] by dissolving the appropriate amount of salt in distilled water and the required pH was adjusted.

1. Tris/HCl buffer at different pH values was prepared as follows:

   Solution A: 0.2 M Tris (2.4228 g tris [hydroxymethyl] aminomethane) in 100 ml of distilled water.

   Solution B: 0.1 N HCl

   Working buffers pH (7.2-9) were prepared by mixing 25 ml of solution A with an appropriate amount of solution B to adjust the required pH, then the volume was made up to 100 ml with distilled water.

2. TEMG buffer (pH 7.4): 0.01 M Tris buffer containing 1.5 mM Na_2-EDTA, 2 mM β-mercaptoethanol and 10% glycerol. The buffer was prepared by an appropriate dilution of the stock solution to 250 ml.

3. Citric acid/phosphate buffer was prepared as follows:

   Solution A: 0.1 M Citric acid (21.01 g $C_6H_8O_7.1H_2O$) in 100 ml distilled water.

Solution B: 0.2 M Disodium phosphate (3.560 g $Na_2HPO_4.2H_2O$) in 100 ml distilled water.

Working buffers pH (2.2–7.8) were prepared by mixing appropriate volumes of solution A and B to reach the required pH in a final volume of 100 ml. The buffer was also contained 1.5 mM Na_2-EDTA, 2mM β-mercaptoethanol and 10% glycerol.

4. Dextran–coated charcoal (DCC) suspension:

This suspension was prepared by dissolving the following compounds: 1.25 g charcoal, 0.625 g dextran T-70 and 0.2 g gelatin in 100 ml of TEMG buffer pH 7.4.

5. Standard unlabeled testosterone solution: stock solution (250 mg/100 ml) was prepared by dissolving an appropriate weight of testosterone compound in a fewest quantity of ethyl alcohol (99-100%), then the volume was completed to a desired volume with TEMG buffer. Working testosterone concentrations were prepared by serial dilution of the stock solution with TEMG.

2.2. Evaluation of some biochemical constituents in sera and tissues of prostatic tumors patients

2.2.1. Determination of testosterone levels in sera of patients with benign and malignant prostatic tumors

Testosterone levels were measured in sera of benign and malignant prostatic tumors patients and healthy individuals were used as controls by radioimmuno assay (RIA). The assay protocol was described in Table (2-2).

Table (2-2): RIA assay protocol of serum testosterone (ng/ml).

	Testosterone standards (ng/ml)							Unknown			
	0	0.2	0.5	1.0	2.5	7.5	20	(1)	(2)	(3)	(4)
Tube No.	1,2	3,4	5,6	7,8	9,10	11,12	13,14	15,16	17,18	19,20	21,22
Standard serum	50	50	50	50	50	50	50	-	-	-	-
Unknown serum	-	-	-	-	-	-	-	50	50	50	50
^{125}I-Testos.	1000	1000	1000	1000	1000	1000	1000	1000	1000	1000	1000
All volumes are in μL											

The test tubes rack was mixed by shaking or by vortexing each tube gently after that all tubes were incubated in a water bath at 37°C for 90 min. Then the tubes were aspirated and counted by γ-counter for one minute [102].

2.2.2. Determination of testosterone levels in crude nuclear fractions of benign and malignant prostatic tumors

The concentrations of testosterone in crude nuclear fractions of benign and malignant prostatic tumors homogenates were determined by the method of radioimmuno assay (RIA) as explained in section (2.2.1), and the assay protocol used was described in Table (2-2).

Note: The crude nuclear fractions of benign and malignant prostatic tumors were prepared as described in section (2.1.6)

2.2.3. Determination of (Fe, Cu, Zn, Ca and Mg) in sera of patients with benign and malignant prostatic tumors

Iron, copper, zinc, calcium and magnesium levels were determined by atomic absorption spectrophotometry [103-105].

The elements were measured using sera diluted (1:4) with deionized water. Iron was estimated at a wavelength of 248.3 nm, copper at 224.8 nm, zinc at 213.9 nm, calcium at 422.7 nm and magnesium at 285.2 nm.

The experiment was performed by the use of Perkin-Elmer type 5000 Atomic Absorption spectrophotometer.

2.3. Binding studies of ^{125}I-testosterone with their receptors in prostatic tumors homogenates

2.3.1. Estimation of total protein content in prostatic tumors homogenates

Total protein content of prostatic tumors homogenate was determined by the method of Lowry et al [106], using bovine serum albumin (BSA) as the standard protein.

Procedure

1. One milliliter of each standard bovine serum albumin (20, 40, 80, 120, 160, 200 µg/ml) was pipetted in a set of duplicate tubes.

2. One milliliter of (1:10) diluted tumor homogenate was also pipetted in a duplicate tubes.

3. Five milliliters of reagent C were added to all assay tubes.

4. The tubes were shaked and allowed to stand at room temperature for 10 min.

5. Half milliliter of reagent D was added to all assay tubes and mixed immediately.

6. The tubes were left at room temperature for 30 min.

7. The absorbance of the blue solution was read at 750 nm against an appropriate blank.

8. The standard curve was obtained by plotting the absorbance against the corresponding concentration of standard protein as shown in Figure (2-1), and used in the determination of the unknown protein concentration of the prostatic tumors homogenates.

Reagents

1. Reagent A: Alkaline sodium carbonate solution (2% Na_2CO_3 in 0.1 N NaOH).

2. Reagent B: Copper sulphate-sodium potassium tartarate solution (0.5% $CuSO4.5H2O$ in 1% Na, K-tartarate).

   This solution was prepared freshly by dissolving 0.1 g of Na, K-tartarate in 10 ml of $CuSO_4.5H_2O$.

3. Reagent C: Alkaline copper solution, this reagent was prepared by mixing 50 ml of reagent A with 1 ml of reagent B.

4. Reagent D: Folin Cio Calteau reagent was prepared by the dilution of the commercial reagent with an equal volume of distilled water on the day of use.

5. Standard bovine serum albumin (stock BSA 0.2 mg/ml): working BSA solutions were prepared by serial dilution of stock solution.

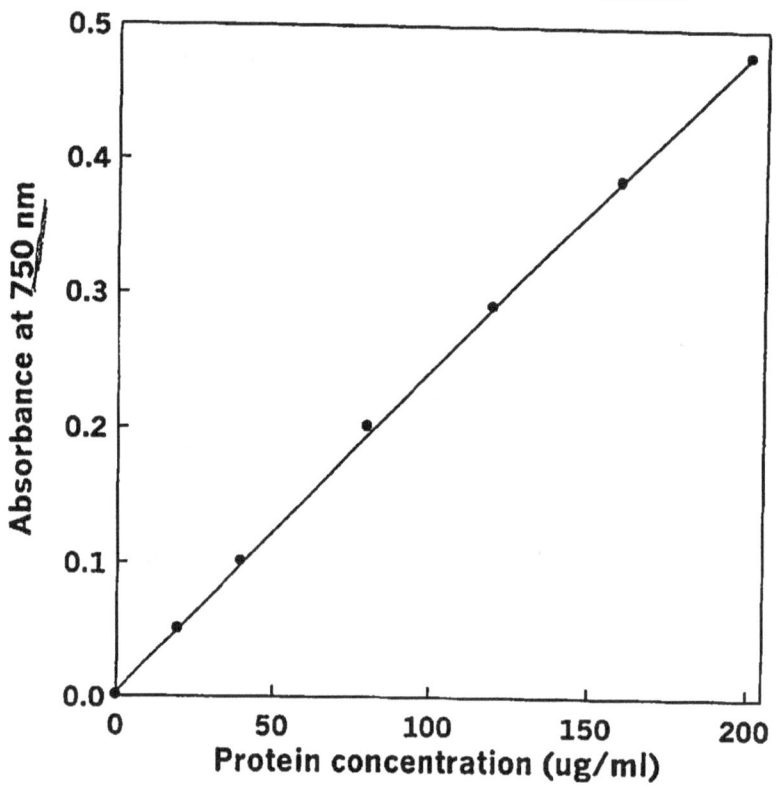

Figure (2-1): The standard curve for protein determination by the Lowry method.

2.3.2. Estimation of DNA content in prostatic tumor homogenate

DNA content of the homogenate was determined by Burton method [107], using calf thymus DNA as a standard.

Procedure

1. One milliliter of each of standard calf thymus DNA (50, 100, 150, 200, 250, 300 μg/ml) was prepared by the dilution of stock solution with 0.5 N HClO$_4$.

2. Half milliliter of crude nuclear fraction was completed to 1 ml with 0.5 N HClO4.

3. Two milliliters of diphenylamine reagent was added to all assay tubes and mixed immediately.

4. The tubes were incubated at 100°C for 10 min, then the tubes were left to cool and the absorbances of blue solutions were read at 600 nm against an appropriate blank.

5. The standard curve was obtained by plotting the absorbance against the corresponding concentration of standard calf thymus DNA as shown in Figure (2-2) and used to determine the unknown content of DNA from the nuclear fractions.

Solutions

1. Diphenylamine reagent (1.5 %)

This reagent was prepared by dissolving 1.5 g of steam-distilled diphenylamine in 100 ml of glacial acetic acid and adding 1.5 ml of concentrated H_2SO_4. The reagent is stored in the dark. On the day it is to be used, 0.1 ml of aqueous acetaldehyde (16 mg/ml) is added for each 20 ml of reagent required.

2. $HClO_4$ (0.5 N)

This solution was prepared by the dilution of 25 ml of 20% $HClO_4$ to 100 ml of distilled water.

3. Standard calf thymus DNA

Stock solution (0.5 mg/ml) was prepared by dissolving 50 mg of calf thymus DNA in 100 ml of 0.5 N $HClO_4$, the solution was heated at 70°C for 30 min. and finally it was cooled and stored at 4°C. The working DNA concentrations were prepared by serial dilution of the stock solution.

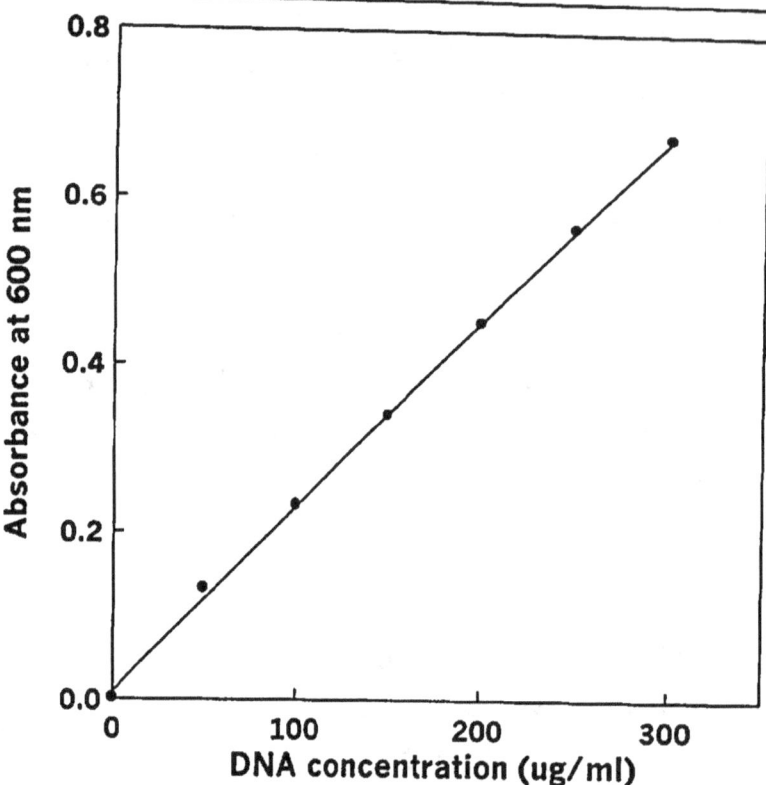

Figure (2-2): The standard curve for DNA determination by Burton method.

2.3.3. Preliminary test of ^{125}I-testosterone binding to its cytosolic and nuclear receptors in human benign and malignant prostatic tumors

Cytosolic and nuclear receptors were evaluated using two sets of duplicate tubes. The first set was carried out to determine the total binding, while the second was used for the estimation of non-specific binding. In order to detect cytosolic receptors 50μL (125 μg protein of BPH or 90 μg protein of PCA) of crude cytosol were incubated with 50 μl (8.7 PM) of ^{125}I-testosterone in duplicate tubes. The volumes of the mixtures were completed to 1 ml with TEMG buffer pH 7.4 and the tubes were incubated for 18 hrs at 4°C. Non-specific binding was accounted for by preparing the same incubation with the addition of 250 fold excess of unlabeled testosterone as a competitor. After incubation, the bound testosterone was estimated by the dextran-coated charcoal method [65]. For this purpose 250μl of dextran-coated charcoal (DCC) were added. The tubes were shaken for 10 min. and centrifuged for 10 min. at 2000 xg. An aliquot of 1 ml was taken from each supernatant and counted by γ-counter.

Crude nuclear receptors were evaluated by the addition of 50 µl (275 µg DNA of BPH or 400 µg DNA of PCA) of crude nuclear fraction to 50 µl (8.7 PM) of ^{125}I-testosterone with and without the addition of 250 fold excess of unlabeled testosterone. The final volume of the mixture was completed with TEMG buffer at pH 7.4 to 1 ml, the mixtures were incubated at 4°C for 18 hrs. During this time the tubes were vortexed several times. At the end of a period of incubation, bound and unbound testosterone were separated by charcoal adsorption with a suspension of dextran-coated charcoal. For this purpose 250µl of dextran-coated charcoal (DCC) were added. The tubes were shaken for 10 min and then centrifuged for 10 min at 2000 xg at 4°C. One milliliter of each supernatant was taken and counted by γ-counter. It represents nuclear bound testosterone.

Solutions

All solutions were prepared as described previously in section (2.1.7).

Calculations

1. The radioactivity in each tube (expressed in cpm) represents the total binding (TB).

2. The radioactivity (expressed in cpm) in the tubes contained ^{125}I-testosterone and excess of unlabeled testosterone represents the non-specific binding (NSB).

3. The specific binding (expressed in cpm) was calculated by subtracting the radioactivity (expressed in cpm) obtained in the presence of unlabeled testosterone from that produced in the absence of unlabeled testosterone.

$$SB (cpm) = TB (cpm) - NSB (cpm)$$

4. The percent of specific binding (SB%) can be calculated from the following formula:

$$SB\% = \frac{SB(cpm)}{Tc(cpm)} \times 100$$

Where: Tc total count of the ^{125}I-testosterone (expressed in cpm) used in each tube.

2.4. Radioreceptor studies of ^{125}I-testosterone binding to its receptors in human benign and malignant prostatic tumors

All the following experiments were carried out with two sets of duplicate tubes. The first one was used to estimate the total binding and the second to estimate the non-specific binding.

2.4.1. The effect of different concentrations of testosterone receptors (DNA or protein) on the binding of ^{125}I-testosterone in prostatic tumor homogenate

Fifty microliters (8.7 PM) of ^{125}I-testosterone were added to 50 µl of increasing amounts (45, 90, 180, 270, 360, 450 µg DNA) of crude benign nuclear fraction and (150, 300, 450, 600, 750 µg DNA) of crude malignant nuclear fraction or (50, 100, 150, 200, 250 µg protein) of crude benign and malignant nuclear fractions in a final volume of 1 ml (completed with TEMG buffer pH 7.4) with and without the addition of 250 fold excess of unlabeled testosterone. At the end of incubation (18 hrs) at 4°C, the bound testosterone was estimated by adding 250 µl of DCC, then the tubes were shaken for 10 min. and centrifuged for 10 min. at 4°C at 2000 xg. One milliliter of each supernatant was taken and counted by γ-counter. It represents the bound hormone.

Solutions

All solutions were prepared as described previously in section (2.1.7)

Calculations

1. The percent of specific binding (SB%) was calculated according to the formula mentioned in section (2.3.3).
2. The percent of specific binding was plotted against the amount of protein and DNA concentration included in each mixture.

2.4.2. The effect of different concentrations of ^{125}I-testosterone on the binding with its receptors in benign and malignant prostatic tumor homogenate

Increasing concentrations (0.87-17.4 PM) of ^{125}I-testosterone was each added to 50µl (200 µg protein or 360 µg DNA) of benign crude nuclear fraction and (150 µg protein or 450 µg DNA) of malignant crude nuclear fraction in the first set of tubes with a final volume of 1 ml (completed with TEMG buffer pH 7.4). The second set of tubes consists of the same reactants plus 250 fold excess of unlabeled testosterone. After incubation for 18 hrs at 4°C, 250 µl of DCC were added in order to estimate the bound testosterone then the tubes were shaken for 10 min and centrifuged for 10 min at 4°C at 2000 xg. One milliliter was taken from each supernatant and counted by γ-counter. It represents the bound testosterone.

Solutions

All solutions were prepared as described previously in section (2.1.7).

Calculations

1. The same mathematical formula mentioned in section (2.3.3) was used to calculate (SB%).
2. The value of (SB%) was plotted against the concentration of ^{125}I-testosterone.

2.4.3. The effect of different pH on the binding of ^{125}I-testosterone to the receptors in prostatic tumor homogenate

Crude nuclear fractions (360 µg of DNA in 50 µl of BPH and 450 µg of DNA in 50µl of PCA) were added to 50 µl (8.7 PM) for benign tumors and 25 µl (4.35 pM) for malignant tumors of ^{125}I-testosterone with and without the addition of 250 fold excess of unlabeled testosterone. The volumes of the mixtures were made up to 1 ml with citric acid/phosphate buffer of different pHs ranging from 7 to 7.6 and with TEMG buffer of different pHs ranging from 7.8 to 9.0. The tubes were incubated at 4°C for 18 hrs. After incubation, the bound testosterone was estimated as mentioned in section (2.3.3).

Solutions

All solutions were prepared as described previously in section (2.1.7).

Calculations

1. The (SB%) was estimated as mentioned in section (2.3.3) at each pH.
2. The percent of specific binding (SB%) was plotted against their corresponding pH.

2.4.4. The Choice of most appropriate incubation time of ^{125}I-testosterone binding to receptors in prostatic tumor homogenate

Fifty microliters (8.7 PM) for benign tumors and 25 µl (4.35 PM) for malignant tumors of ^{125}I-testosterone were added to 50 µl (360 µg of DNA of benign tumors and 450 µg of DNA of malignant tumors) of crude nuclear fraction in a final volume of 1 ml (completed with TEMG buffer pH 7.8 for benign tumors and pH 8.5 for malignant tumors) with and without the addition of 250 fold excess of unlabeled testosterone. The tubes were incubated at 4°C. At certain time intervals (2,4,6,8,10,12,14,16,18,20 hrs) two tubes from each set were taken and the bound hormone was estimated as mentioned in section (2.3.3).

Solutions

All solutions were prepared as described previously in section (2.1.7).

Calculations

1. The (SB%) was estimated as mentioned in section (2.3.3) at each incubation time.
2. The percent of specific binding (SB%) was plotted against their corresponding time.

2.4.5.Temperature dependency of the binding between ^{125}I-testosterone and their receptors in prostatic tumors

Fifty microliters (8.7 PM) for benign tumors and 25 µl (4.35 PM) for malignant tumors of ^{125}I-testosterone was added to 50 µl (360 µg of DNA of benign tumors and 450 µg of DNA of malignant tumors) of crude nuclear fraction in a final volume of 1 ml (completed with TEMG buffer pH 7.8 for benign tumors and pH 8.5 for malignant tumors) with and without the addition of 250 fold excess of unlabeled testosterone. After incubation for 16 hrs (benign and malignant tumors) at 4°C, the bound testosterone was estimated as mentioned in sections (2.3.3) and (2.4.1).

The experiment was performed at different temperatures (4, 10, 25, 37, 45 and 55°C).

Solutions

All solutions were prepared as described previously in section (2.1.7).

Calculations

1. The percent of specific binding (SB%) was estimated according to section (2.3.3) at each temperature.
2. The percents of specific binding (SB%) were plotted against the different temperatures of incubation.

2.4.6. The effect of different halides on the binding of ^{125}I-testosterone to its receptors in prostatic tumors

Fifty microliters of crude nuclear fractions (360 µg of DNA of benign tumors and 450 µg of DNA of malignant tumors) were incubated with 50µl (8.7 PM) for benign tumors or with 25 µl (4.35 PM) for malignant tumors of ^{125}I-testosterone with and without the addition of 250 fold excess of unlabeled testosterone in a final volume of 1 ml (completed with TEMG buffer pH 7.8 for benign tumors and pH 8.5 for malignant tumors containing 0.1 M of each of the following halides: NaF, NaCl and NaI). The tubes were incubated for 16 hrs at

37°C (benign tumors) and at 45°C (malignant tumors), then the bound testosterone was estimated as mentioned in section (2.3.3).

The control was used without the addition of any halide.

Solutions

Halides solutions were prepared in concentration of 0.1 M in TEMG buffer pH 7.8 (benign tumors) and pH 8.5 (malignant tumors), 1.0497 gm of NaF in 250 ml of TEMG buffer, 1.461 gm of NaCl in 250 ml of TEMG buffer, 3.750 gm NaI in 250 ml of TEMG buffer.

Calculations

1. The (SB%) was estimated according to section (2.3.3) at each halide.
2. The percent of specific binding (SB%) was plotted against each type of halide.

2.4.7. The effect of monovalent salts on the binding of ^{125}I-testosterone to its receptors in benign and malignant human prostate tumors

The experiment was performed at optimum conditions (temperature, time, pH, ^{125}I-testosterone and DNA concentration) as mentioned in section (2.4.6) with one exception that the reaction mixtures were completed to 1 ml with TEMG buffer containing 0.1 M of different monovalent salts (NH_4Cl, KCl, LiCl, CsCl and NaCl). The bound hormone was estimated as mentioned in section (2.3.3). The control was used without the addition of any salt.

Solutions

Monovalent salts were prepared in 0.1 M in TEMG buffer (pH 7.8 for benign tumors and pH 8.5 for malignant tumors), 1.8640 gm of KCl in 250 ml of TEMG buffer, 1.3372 g of NH_4Cl in 250 ml of TEMG buffer, 4.209 gm of CsCl in 250 ml of TEMG buffer, 1.5102 gm of LiCl in 250 ml of TEMG buffer.

Calculations

1. The (SB%) was estimated according to section (2.3.3) for each salt.
2. The percent of specific binding (SB%) was plotted against each salt type.

2.4.8. The effect of divalent cations on the binding of ^{125}I-testosterone with its receptors in prostatic tumor homogenate

To evaluate the effect of divalent cations on the testosterone binding with its human prostatic receptors, the experiment was carried out at optimum conditions of time, temperature, pH, ^{125}I-testosterone and DNA concentration with one exception that the reaction mixtures were completed to 1 ml with TEMG buffer containing 25 mM of each of the following salts: $MgCl_2.6H_2O$, $MnCl_2.4H_2O$, $CuSO_4.5H_2O$, $CaCl_2$, $ZnCl_2$ and $ZnSO_4$.

The bound testosterone was estimated as mentioned in section (2.3.3). The control was used without the addition of any salt.

Solutions

The stock solutions (25 mM) of divalent salts were prepared as the following: 1.2706 gm $MgCl_2$ in 250 ml of TEMG buffer, 1.2369 gm $MnCl_2$ in 250 ml of TEMG buffer, 1.5597gm $CuSO_4$ in 250 ml of TEMG buffer, 0.6936 gm $CaCl_2$ in 250 ml of TEMG buffer, 0.8518 gm $ZnCl_2$ in 250 ml of TEMG buffer and 1.7971 gm $ZnSO_4$ in 250 ml of TEMG buffer.

Calculations

1. The (SB%) was estimated according to section (2.3.3) for each salt.

2. The percent of specific binding (SB%) was plotted against each salt type.

2.4.9. The choice of most appropriate concentration of β-mercaptoethanol for the binding of ^{125}I-testosterone with their receptors in benign and malignant prostatic tumors

The experiment was carried out at optimum conditions of time, temperature, pH, ^{125}I-testosterone and DNA concentration with an exception that the reaction mixtures were completed to 1 ml with TEMG buffer containing β-mercaptoethanol ranging in their concentrations from 0.5 to 20 mM.

The bound testosterone was estimated as mentioned in section (2.3.3). The control in this experiment was used without the addition of the salt.

Solutions

The different β-mercaptoethanol concentrations were prepared by appropriate serial dilution starting with the stock solution (36 mM).

Calculations

1. The (SB%) was estimated as mentioned in section (2.3.3).
2. The percent of specific binding (SB%) values were plotted against the concentrations of β-mercaptoethanol.

2.4.10. The effect of urea on the binding of ^{125}I-testosterone with its crude nuclear receptors in benign and malignant prostatic tumors

The experiment was carried out at optimum conditions of time, temperature, pH, ^{125}I-testosterone and DNA concentration with an exception that the reaction mixtures were completed to 1 ml with TEMG buffer containing urea ranging in their concentrations from 0.1 to 4 M. The bound testosterone was estimated as mentioned in section (2.3.3). The control in this experiment was used without the addition of urea.

Solutions

1. The stock urea solution (8M) was prepared by dissolving 48 g in 100 ml of TEMG buffer pH 7.8 (benign tumor) and pH 8.5 (malignant tumors).

2. Various solutions of urea ranging in their molar concentrations from 0.1 to 4 M were prepared by the serial dilution of the stock.

Calculations

1. The (SB%) was estimated using the same mathematical formula of section (2.3.3) at each urea concentration.

2. The values of (SB%) were plotted versus the corresponding molar concentrations of urea solutions.

2.4.11. The effect of polyethylene glycol on the binding of ^{125}I-testosterone with their human prostatic tumors receptors

The experiment was carried out at optimum conditions as mentioned in section (2.4.6) with an exception that the reaction mixtures were completed to 1 ml with TEMG buffer containing various percents of polyethylene glycol (PEG-6000) ranging from 1 to 6%. The bound testosterone was estimated as mentioned in section (2.3.3). The control used in this experiment was without the addition of PEG.

Solutions

The stock solution of PEG-6000 (10%) was prepared by dissolving 10 g of PEG in 100 ml of TEMG buffer (pH 7.8 for benign tumors and pH 8.5 for malignant tumors); 1,2,3,4,5 and 6% of PEG solutions were prepared by an appropriate serial dilution of the stock solution.

Calculations

1. The (SB%) was estimated as mentioned in section (2.3.3) at each PEG percent.

2. The (SB%) values were plotted against PEG percents.

2.4.12. The effect of molybdate ion on the binding of ^{125}I-testosterone with its receptors in benign and malignant prostatic tumors

To evaluate the effect of molybdate ion on the binding, the experiment was carried out at optimum conditions as mentioned in section (2.4.6) with an exception that the reaction mixtures were completed to 1 ml with TEMG buffer containing different molybdate concentrations 0.5, 1, 1.5, 2.5 3.5 and 4.5 mM. The bound testosterone was estimated as mentioned in section (2.3.3). The control used in this experiment was without the addition of molybdate.

Solutions

The stock solution of ammonium molybdate $(NH_4)_6Mo_7.O_{24}.4H_2O$ (5mM) was prepared by dissolving 0.6179 g in 100 ml of TEMG buffer, 0.5, 1, 1.5, 2.5, 3.5 and 4.5 mM were prepared by an appropriate serial dilution of the stock solution.

Calculations

1. The (SB%) was estimated as mentioned in section (2.3.3).
2. The (SB%) values were plotted against the molybdate ion concentrations.

2.4.13. The effect of N-bromosuccinimide (NBS) on the binding of ^{125}I-testosterone with its receptors in benign and malignant prostatic tumors

The experiment was carried out at optimum conditions of time, temperature, pH, ^{125}I-testosterone and DNA concentration as mentioned in section (2.4.6) with an exception that the reaction mixtures were completed to 1 ml with TEMG buffer containing different concentrations of NBS. The bound testosterone was estimated as mentioned in section (2.3.3). The control used in this experiment was without the addition of NBS.

Solutions

Stock NBS (50mM) was prepared by dissolving 0.8899 g of NBS in 100 ml of TEMG buffer. Various solutions of NBS ranging in their concentrations from 5 to 40 mM were prepared by an appropriate serial dilution of the stock solution.

Calculations

1. The (SB%) was estimated as mentioned in section (2.3.3) at each NBS concentration.
2. The (SB%) was plotted against their corresponding NBS concentration.

2.4.14. Stability of ^{125}I-testosterone-receptor complex

This experiment was carried out at the optimum conditions of ^{125}I-testosterone and DNA concentration, time, temperature and pH, in order to investigate the effect of temperature on ^{125}I-testosterone–receptor complex properties. The experiment was performed as described previously in section (2.4.6). The exception of this experiment was that the reaction mixtures were completed to 1 ml with TEMG (b) buffer pH 7.8 for benign tumors and with TEMG (m) buffer pH 8.5 for malignant tumors. The bound testosterone (testosterone-receptor complex) was reincubated at different temperatures (0,4,10,25°C). Between 0 and 1.5 hrs the remaining bound testosterone in each tube was measured as described in section (2.3.3).

Solutions

TEMG (b) buffer (pH 7.8)

0.01 M tris containing 1.5 mM Na$_2$-EDTA, 2.5 mM β-mercaptoethanol, 10% glycerol, 0.1 M NaCl and 25 mM CaCl$_2$.

TEMG (m) buffer (pH 8.5)

0.01 M tris containing 1.5 mM Na$_2$-EDTA, 10 mM β-mercaptoethanol, 10% glycerol, 0.1 M NaCl and 25 mM MgCl$_2$.

Calculations

1. The relative specific binding percent (RSB%) was estimated from the following formula:

$$RSB\% \frac{(SB)_t}{(SB)_o} \times 100$$

Where:

$(SB)_t$ = specific binding (cpm) of ^{125}I-testosterone at time (t) of reincubation.

$(SB)_o$ = specific binding (cpm) of ^{125}I-testosterone at time zero of reincubation.

2. The percent of relative specific binding (RSB%) was plotted against the time of reincubation.

2.4.15. Competitive effect of different concentrations of unlabeled testosterone, estrone and estriol on the binding of ^{125}I-testosterone to its receptors in human prostatic tumors

The experiment was carried out at the optimum conditions as described in section (2.4.14) with an exception that it was performed with and without the addition of increasing concentrations (5-500 nM) of unlabeled testosterone. The bound testosterone was measured as described in section (2.3.3). The experiment was repeated with increasing concentrations of unlabeled estrone and estriol.

Solutions

TEMG (b) and TEMG (m) buffers were prepared as described previously in section (2.4.14).

Calculations

1. The percent of relative specific binding (RSB%) was estimated from the following formula:

$$RSB\% = \frac{\text{Specific binding of }^{125}\text{I} - \text{testosterone in the prsence of a compétitor}}{\text{Specific binding of }^{125}\text{I} - \text{testosterone in the absence of a competitor}} \times 100$$

2. The percents of relative specific binding (%RSB) were plotted against the different concentrations of competitors (testosterone, estrone and estriol).

3. For the purpose of comparison [108], it was found that the following method was very practical in analyzing the results of the competition experiments.

   In the "receptor binding assay":

$$Y = \frac{\text{Pr otein} - \text{bound cpm in the prsence of a competitor}}{\text{Pr otein} - \text{bound cpm in the absence of a competitor}}$$

   and in the "nuclear retention assay":

$$Y = \frac{\text{Nuclear} - \text{bound cpm in the prsence of a competitor}}{\text{Nuclear} - \text{bound cpm in the absence of a competitor}}$$

   Then

$$Y = \frac{[^{125}\text{I--testosterone}]}{[^{125}\text{I--testosterone}] + a\,[\text{competitor}]}$$

Where:

$[^{125}\text{I-testosterone}]$ and $[\text{competitor}]$ are, respectively, the concentrations of ^{125}I-testosterone and the competitor in the assay system and (a) is a factor (competition index: CI) that is characteristic of a competing steroid. This factor can be used to compare the relative ability of various steroids to compete with testosterone for nuclear receptor binding or for nuclear retention by plotting $\dfrac{1}{Y}$ as a function of $\dfrac{[\text{competitor}]}{[^{125}\text{I} - \text{testost.}]}$, (a) was obtained from the slope. The plot is called "RC (relative competition) plot". Theoretically, a is 1 for non radioactive testosterone.

4. The relative competition index (RCI) for a competitor is then calculated from:

$$RCI_{comp.} = \frac{a_{comp.}}{a_{testost.}}$$

2.5. Kinetics and thermodynamics of the interaction of testosterone with its nuclear receptors

2.5.1. The time course of ^{125}I-testosterone binding to its nuclear receptors in benign and malignant prostatic tumors

1. At zero time, the experiment was carried out at the optimum conditions of pH, ^{125}I-testosterone and DNA concentration. Incubation was carried out for several time intervals (2,4,6,8,10,12,14,16,18,20 and 22 hrs).

2. After each time interval, the bound testosterone was estimated as described previously in section (2.3.3).

3. Parallel experiments were performed to determine the amount of non-specific binding.

4. To determine the time course of the association of ^{125}I-testosterone with its receptors in benign and malignant prostatic tumors at different temperatures, the above experiment was performed at five temperatures, i.e., 4,10,25,37 and 45°C.

Solutions

All solutions were prepared as described previously in sections (2.4.14) and (2.1.7.).

Calculations

1. The value of ^{125}I-testosterone bound specifically in (picomole of ^{125}I-testosterone per mg of protein or DNA) was calculated according to the following formula:

$$\begin{pmatrix} \text{The value of specifically} \\ \text{bound } ^{125}\text{I} - \text{testosterone} \\ \text{(pmole / mg protein or DNA)} \end{pmatrix} = \frac{\begin{pmatrix} \text{Specifically bound} \\ ^{125}\text{I} - \text{testosterone in (PM)} \end{pmatrix} \times \begin{pmatrix} \text{Incubation volume in} \\ \text{(Liter)} \end{pmatrix}}{\text{mgs of protein or DNA in incubation medium}}$$

$$\begin{pmatrix} \text{Specifically bound} \\ ^{125}\text{I} - \text{testosterone} \\ \text{(PM)} \end{pmatrix} = \frac{(\text{Total binding (cpm)}) - (\text{Non} - \text{specific binding (cpm)})}{\text{Total counts (cpm)}} \times \begin{pmatrix} \text{Total} \\ \text{concentration of} \\ ^{125}\text{I} - \text{testosterone} \\ \text{in incubation} \\ \text{medium} \end{pmatrix}$$

$$\begin{pmatrix} \text{The percent of} \\ \text{specific binding} \\ \text{(SB\%)} \end{pmatrix} = \left[\frac{(\text{Total binding (cpm)}) - (\text{Non} - \text{specific binding (cpm)})}{\text{Total counts (cpm) of } ^{125}\text{I} - \text{testosterone used in each tube}} \right] \times 100$$

2. The plot of the values of SB% or the values of ^{125}I-testosterone specifically bound in (PM) against the time intervals yielded the time course curve for the association of the ^{125}I-testosterone with its receptors in the human prostate gland.

2.5.2. Determination of the concentration of testosterone receptors and the affinity constant of ^{125}I-testosterone association with its receptors in benign and malignant prostatic tumors

Crude nuclear testosterone receptors were measured by the addition of increasing concentrations (1.742-26.13 PM) of ^{125}I-testosterone to 50 µl (360 µg DNA of crude benign nuclear fraction and 450 µg DNA of crude malignant nuclear fraction) with and without the addition of 250 fold excess of unlabeled testosterone in a final volume of 1 ml (completed with TEMG (b) buffer pH 7.8 for benign tumors and with TEMG (m) buffer pH 8.5 for malignant tumors). The tubes were incubated for 16 hrs at 37°C (benign tumors) and at 45°C (malignant tumors) in order to attain an equilibrium state. The bound testosterone was estimated as mentioned in section (2.3.3). All the previous steps of this experiment were performed at different temperatures. The time of incubation needed to get the equilibrium state at each temperature was obtained from the related time course pattern.

Solutions

All solutions were prepared as described previously in sections (2.4.14) and (2.1.7).

Calculations

1. The values of ^{125}I-testosterone which is bound specifically in picomolar were calculated using the following formula:

$$B = \frac{\text{Total binding} - \text{Non} - \text{specific binding}}{\text{Total count}} \times \text{concentration of } ^{125}\text{I} - \text{testosterone(PM)}$$

in each assay tube

2. The concentration of receptors and the affinity constant were determined according to Scatchard equation [109,110]:

$$\frac{B}{F} = \frac{1}{k_d}(B_{max} - B)$$

$$k_a = \frac{1}{k_d}$$

Where:

B: The concentration of specifically bound testosterone.

F: The concentration of free testosterone.

K_a: The affinity constant.

B_{max}: The maximal binding capacity.

K_d: The dissociation constant.

3. The B/F values were plotted against the values of the B, the receptor concentration and the affinity constant were calculated from the x-axis and the slope of the straight line respectively.

2.5.3. Estimation of Hill coefficients (n) of nuclear receptors of benign and malignant human prostatic tumors

To assess the cooperativity of the binding, the experiment was performed as described in section (2.5.2) using 50 µl of crude nuclear fraction (360 µg DNA of benign tumors and 450 µg DNA of malignant tumors). The bound testosterone was measured as mentioned in section (2.3.3).

Solutions

All solutions were prepared as described previously in sections (2.4.14) and (2.1.7).

Calculations

1. The values of ^{125}I-testosterone bound specifically in (PM) which was represented by B were calculated from the mathematical formula mentioned in section (2.5.1) and (2.5.2).

2. The Hill coefficients were obtained using the following equation, known as logarithmic form of the Hill-equation [110]:

$$\log\left[\frac{B}{B_{max} - B}\right] = n\log F - \log k'$$

Where:

F: Free ^{125}I-testosterone concentration in the incubation medium.

n: Hill coefficient.

and k': Constant comprising the interaction factors and the intrinsic dissociation constant ·

3. $\log\left[\dfrac{B}{B_{max} - B}\right]$ was plotted against the log F. The slope of the straight line gives the Hill coefficient (n) value.

2.5.4. The thermodynamics of ^{125}I-testosterone interaction with its receptors in benign and malignant prostatic tumors

Fifty microliters of prostatic tumor homogenate (360 µg DNA of benign tumors and 450 µg DNA of malignant tumors) was incubated with 8.7 PM of ^{125}I-testosterone at 37°C for 16 hrs (for benign tumors) and incubated with 4.35 PM of ^{125}I-testosterone at 45°C for 16 hrs (for malignant tumors). The final volume (1 ml) was made up by adding the assay buffer (TEMG (b) pH 7.8 for benign tumors and TEMG (m) pH 8.5 for malignant tumors). The steps 2,3 and 4 of the experiment (2.5.1) were carried out for several time intervals (2, 4, 6, 8, 10, 12, 14, 16, 18, 20 and 22 hrs).

Solutions

All solutions were prepared as described previously in sections (2.4.14) and (2.1.7).

Calculations

1. The thermodynamic parameters of standard state were obtained from Van't Hoff plot, the values of the natural logarithm of equilibrium constant (affinity constant k_a) obtained at different temperatures were plotted against the reciprocal values of absolute temperature in Kelvin (1/T), according to the following equation:

$$\ln k_a = \frac{\Delta S^\circ}{R} - \frac{\Delta H^\circ}{RT}$$

Where:

ΔH°: The enthalpy change of the standard state,

ΔS°: The entropy change of the standard state,

R: The gas constant (8.3144 J.mol^{-1}.K^{-1}).

ΔH° value was obtained from the slope of the linear relationship of the plot. The change in Gibbs free energy of the standard state (ΔG°) was calculated from the following equation:

$$\Delta G^\circ = -RT \ln k_a$$

In addition, the standard state entropy change (ΔS^o) was calculated from the following formula:

$$\Delta S^o = \frac{\left(\Delta H^o - \Delta G^o\right)}{T}$$

2. The thermodynamic parameters of the transition state were estimated from Arrhenius plot of ln k_{+1} versus (1/T) which gives a linear relationship according to the following equation:

$$\ln k_{+1} = \ln A - \left(\frac{E_a}{RT}\right)$$

Where:

A: The Arrhenius constant,

E_a: The activation energy,

R: The gas constant, and

T: Absolute temperature.

The activation energy of the binding reaction was calculated from the slope of the straight line. The enthalpy of the transition state (ΔH^*) was determined from:

$$\Delta H^* = E_a - RT$$

The transition state of free energy (ΔG^*) was calculated from the following equation;

$$\Delta G^* = -RT \ln k_{+1} + RT \ln\left(\frac{kT}{h}\right)$$

Where:

k: is Boltzmann constant (1.38×10^{-23} J.deg^{-1}).

h: is Plank constant (0.662×10^{-33} J.sec^{-1}).

The change in entropy of the transition state (ΔS^*) was calculated from the following formula:

$$\Delta S^* = \frac{\left(\Delta H^* - \Delta G^*\right)}{T}$$

Temperature coefficient (Q_{10}) was also determined from the integrated form of the Arrhenius equation [110,111]:

$$\ln Q_{10} = \frac{E_a}{R}\left(\frac{10}{T_2 T_1}\right)$$

2.6. Purification of nuclear testosterone receptors using gel filtration technique

2.6.1. Gel preparation and column packing [112,113]

The gel was allowed to swell in excess of buffer (A) pH 7.8 (50 ml buffer/g of gel) and left to stand for three days (72 hrs) at room temperature without stirring, the gel slurry were degassed by suction for 1 hr, then the swollen gel was poured carefully into a vertical glass-column down the wall using a glass-rod. After the gel has settled the column was equilibrated with buffer (A) pH 7.8 for 24 hrs with the dimension of (0.7 × 28 cm).

2.6.2. Void volume (V_o) determination

The void volume of the column was estimated using blue dextran 2000 with concentration of 2 mg/ml dissolved in buffer (A) pH 7.8, 0.5 ml of blue dextran solution was applied to the column carefully, then elution was carried out with the same buffer using a flow rate of 5 ml/hr. Fractions of 1 ml were collected and their absorbances were measured at 600 nm. The volume of the buffer that required to elute the blue dextran represents the void volume (6 ml) of the column.

2.6.3. The preparation of nuclear salt extracts

The frozen tissues were weighed, pulverized finely with a scalpel in Petri dish standing on ice bath, and then homogenized at 4°C in TEMG (b) buffer solution with a ratio of 1:5 (weight : volume) using a manual homogenizer. The homogenate was filtered through four layers of nylon gauze to remove tissue clumps and fibers of connective tissues. The filtrate fluid was transferred by a Pasteur pipette to low-speed centrifuge tubes and prepare a crude nuclear pellet by centrifugation at 2000 xg for 15 min. The supernatant was decanted, and the pellet was resuspended in 10 volumes of TEMG (b)-NaCl buffer pH 7.8 for 15 min. Nuclei were allowed to swell at 4°C for 30 min in the same buffer. The nuclei were then ruptured by exposing them to sonic waves for forty .30 seconds intervals. The tubes were kept immersed in ice during the entire procedure. Sonically ruptured nuclei solution was then sedimented in a refrigerated centrifuge at 2000 xg for 60 min. The supernatant was then used as a source of nuclear testosterone receptors [65,114,115].

2.6.4. Purification procedure

Half milliliter of the nuclear salt extract (3.5 mg protein) was applied to the surface of sephadex G-200 column (0.7 × 28 cm) equilibrated with buffer (A). The sample was eluted using the same buffer, fractions of 1 ml were collected at a flow rate of 5 ml/hr. The absorbances of the fractions collected were measured at 280 nm and the protein contents were determined by the method of Lowry et al [106].

2.6.5. The preliminary test of the binding of ^{125}I-testosterone to the purified fractions separated by gel filtration

Fifty microliters of purified fractions were added to 100 µl (17.42 PM) of ^{125}I-testosterone with and without the addition of 250 fold excess of unlabeled testosterone in a final volume of 1 ml completed with TEMG (b) buffer. The tubes were incubated for 16 hrs at 37°C, the bound testosterone was measured as described in section (2.3.3).

2.6.6. Dialysis for concentration

The fractions that contained high levels of testosterone receptors were pooled and concentrated by dialyzing against sucrose at 4°C for 30 min to get the needed concentration.

Solutions

Buffer (A): TEMG (b) buffer pH 7.8 containing 0.02 % sodium azide.

TEMG (b)-NaCl buffer: TEMG (b) buffer pH 7.8 containing 1M-NaCl.

TEMG (b) buffer pH 7.8: was prepared as described previously in section (2.4.14).

Calculations

1. The dimensions of the column were chosen according to the following equations [112]:

$$\text{Diameter (cm)} = \sqrt[3]{\frac{m}{10}},$$

Where:

m is the amount of protein in mg.

Length (cm) = 30 × diameter

In view of the results of such calculation, a 0.7 × 28 cm, column has been used.

2. The values of SB% for the eluted fractions were calculated in the same method as that of the previous experiments.

3. The values of SB% and absorbances at 280 nm were plotted against the fraction number.

4. The purification fold for each testosterone receptor for benign and malignant human prostatic tumors was estimated from the following formula:

$$\text{Purification fold} = \frac{\text{Specific binding of purified receptor (fmole / mg prot.)}}{\text{Specific binding of crude receptor (fmole / mg prot.)}}$$

2.7. The choice of most appropriate conditions of ^{125}I-testosterone binding to its purified nuclear receptors

2.7.1. The effect of different purified testosterone receptor concentration on the binding in human prostatic homogenate

One hundred microliters (17.42 PM) of ^{125}I-testosterone were added to 50 μl of increasing amounts (50, 100, 150, 200, 250 μg) of purified nuclear testosterone receptors (BI and BII from benign tumors, MI and MII from malignant tumors) in a final volume of 0.6 ml completed with TEMG buffer pH 7.8 with and without the addition of 250 fold excess of unlabeled testosterone. At the end of incubation (16 hrs) at 37°C, the bound testosterone was estimated by adding 200 μl of DCC, then the tubes were shaken for 10 min and centrifuged at 2000 xg for 10 min at 4°C. Six hundred microliters was taken from each supernatant and counted by γ-counter. It represents the bound testosterone.

Solutions

All solutions were prepared as described previously in sections (2.4.14) and (2.1.7).

Calculations

1. The (SB%) value for each protein concentration was calculated in the same method as that of the previous experiments.
2. The values of (SB%) were plotted against protein concentrations for each purified receptor.

2.7.2. The choice of most appropriate ^{125}I-testosterone concentration for the binding with its purified nuclear receptors in human benign and malignant prostatic tumors

Increasing concentrations (28.998-87 PM) of ^{125}I-testosterone was each added to 50 µl (250 µg BI and MI-protein, 200 µg BII-protein, 150 µg MII-protein) in the first set of tubes with a final volume of 0.6 ml completed with TEMG buffer pH 7.8. The second set of tubes consists of the same reactants plus 250 fold excess of unlabeled testosterone. After incubation for 16 hrs at 37°, the bound testosterone was estimated as mentioned in section (2.7.1).

Solutions

All solutions were prepared as described previously in sections (2.4.14) and (2.1.7).

Calculations

1. The (SB%) was estimated as mentioned in section (2.3.3) at each testosterone concentration.
2. The (SB%) was plotted against testosterone concentration.

2.7.3. The effect of pH on the binding of ^{125}I-testosterone to its purified nuclear receptors from human benign and malignant prostatic tumors

Fifty microliters of purified nuclear fractions (250 μg BI and MI-protein, 200 μg BII-protein, 150 μg MII-protein) were added to 150 μl (43.5 PM) for MII purified fraction and to 200 μl (57.997 PM) for BI, BII and MI purified fractions of ^{125}I-testosterone with and without the addition of 250 fold excess of unlabeled testosterone. The volumes of the mixtures were made up to 0.6 ml with TEMG buffer of different pHs ranging from 7.8 to 9.5 and with citric acid/phosphate buffer of pHs ranging from 6.4 to 7.8. The tubes were incubated at 37°C for 16 hrs. After the incubation, the bound testosterone was estimated as mentioned in section (2.7.1).

Solutions

TEMG buffer with different pH required was prepared as described previously in sections (2.4.14) and (2.1.7).

Citric acid-phosphate buffer was prepared as described previously in section (2.1.7).

Calculations

1. The (SB%) was estimated as mentioned in section (2.3.3) at each pH.
2. The (SB%) was plotted against the corresponding pH.

2.7.4. The effect of incubation time on the binding of ^{125}I-testosterone to its purified nuclear receptors in human benign and malignant prostatic tumors

Fifty microliters of purified nuclear fraction (250 μg BI and MI-protein, 200 μg BII-protein, 150 μg MII-protein) were added to 43.5 PM of ^{125}I-testosterone for MII purified fraction and to 57.997 PM for BI, BII and MI purified fractions with and without the addition of 250 fold excess of unlabeled testosterone. The volumes of the mixtures were completed to 0.6 ml with TEMG buffer (pH 7.8 for

BI and MII fractions, pH 8.6 for BII fraction) and with citric acid–phosphate buffer (pH 7 for MI fraction). The tubes were incubated at 37°C for different time intervals (1,2,4,6,10 and 14 hrs). At the end of incubation, the bound testosterone was estimated as described in section (2.7.1).

Solutions

All solutions were prepared as described previously in section (2.7.3).

Calculations

1. The percent of specific binding (SB%) was determined according to section (2.3.3) at each time.

2. The (SB%) values were plotted against the different times of incubation.

2.7.5. Temperature dependency of testosterone binding to its purified nuclear receptors in human prostatic tumors

The experiment was carried out at the optimum conditions of each purified receptor of pH, ^{125}I-testosterone concentration and protein concentration as described in section (2.7.4). The tubes were incubated for (2hrs for BI fraction, 6hrs for BII and MI fractions and 14 hr for MII fraction). The experiment was performed at different temperatures (4,10,25,37 and 45°C), the bound testosterone was estimated as mentioned in section (2.7.1).

Solutions

All solutions were prepared as described previously in section (2.7.3).

Calculations

1. The (SB%) was determined as mentioned in section (2.3.3) at each temperature.

2. The (SB%) values were plotted against the different temperatures of incubation.

2.7.6. The effect of anticancer drugs on the binding of ^{125}I-testosterone to its purified nuclear receptors in human benign and malignant prostatic tumors

The experiment was carried out at the optimum conditions used in section (2.7.5).

Fifty microliters of 10% of each anticancer drug (cisplatin, vincristine sulfate, 5-fluorouracil and cyclophosphamide) was added to incubation mixtures of the different fractions of purified nuclear receptors. Bound testosterone was measured by a method described in section (2.7.1).

Calculations

1. The relative activity percent (a%) was calculated as follows [110]:

$$a\% = \frac{(SB\%)_i}{(SB\%)_o} \times 100$$

Where:

$(SB\%)_i$: The specific binding percent of ^{125}I-testosterone in the presence of a drug.

and $(SB\%)_o$: The specific binding percent of ^{125}I-testosterone in the absence of a drug.

2. The inhibition percent (i %) for each purified nuclear testosterone receptor with each drug used was estimated from the following relation [110]:

i % = 100 – a%.

2.8. The kinetics and thermodynamics of the interaction of testosterone with its purified nuclear receptors in human benign and malignant prostatic tumors

2.8.1. The time course of the ^{125}I-testosterone association with its purified nuclear receptors

1. At zero time, the experiment was carried out at the optimum conditions of pH, protein and ^{125}I-testosterone concentration for all purified fractions (BI, BII, MI and MII) as described in section (2.7.4).

2. The tubes were incubated at 4°C for several time intervals (1,2,4,6,10,14 hrs).

3. After incubation, the bound testosterone was estimated as mentioned in section (2.7.1).

4. Parallel experiments were performed to determine the amounts of non-specific binding.

5. To determine the time course of the association of ^{125}I-testosterone with its purified receptors at different temperatures, the above experiment was performed at five temperatures (4,10,25,37 and 45°C) for each purified fraction.

Solutions

All solutions were prepared as described previously in section (2.7.3).

Calculations

The same mathematical formulae mentioned in section (2.5.1) were used.

2.8.2. Determination of the concentration of purified nuclear testosterone receptors and the affinity constant of testosterone association with its purified nuclear receptors in human benign and malignant prostatic tumors

Purified nuclear receptors were measured by using of increasing concentrations (8.71-34.84 PM) of ^{125}I-testosterone. The experiment was carried out at the optimum conditions of protein concentration and pH for each purified fraction as mentioned in section (2.7.5). It was performed at different temperatures (4,10,25,37 and 45°C). The bound testosterone was estimated as mentioned in section (2.7.1). The times of incubation needed to get the equilibrium state of different fractions at each temperature were obtained from the related time course patterns.

Solutions

All solutions were prepared as described previously in section (2.7.3).

Calculations

The same mathematical formulae mentioned in section (2.5.2) were used.

2.8.3. Estimation of Hill coefficients (n) of purified nuclear testosterone receptors

The experiment was performed as described in sections (2.8.2) and (2.5.3) using 50 µl of purified nuclear fractions (250 µg BI, MI-protein, 200 µg BII-protein and 150 µg MII-protein) at 37°C and bound testosterone was measured by the method described in section (2.7.1).

Solutions

All solutions were prepared as described previously in section (2.7.3).

Calculations

All mathematical formulae and equations were mentioned in section (2.5.3).

2.8.4 The thermodynamics of the association of testosterone with its purified nuclear receptors in human benign and malignant prostatic tumors

The experiment was carried out at the optimum conditions of pH, ^{125}I-testosterone and protein concentration for all purified fractions as described in section (2.7.4). The steps 2,3 and 4 of the experiment (2.8.1) were carried out at different temperatures (4,10,25,37,and 45°C).

Solutions

All solutions were prepared as described previously in section (2.7.3).

Calculations

The same mathematical equations and relations mentioned in section (2.5.4) were used.

2.9. Spectroscopic studies of different purified forms of testosterone receptors

2.9.1. The U.V. spectra of purified nuclear testosterone receptors in human benign and malignant prostatic tumors

One hundred microliters (350 µg protein) of each purified nuclear receptor was completed to 0.5 ml with distilled water pH 7.4, then placed in a 0.5cm cuvette in sample beam and the absorption spectrum was immediately measured against the adjusted pH .... distilled water as a reference.

2.9.2. Factors affecting the absorption properties of purified nuclear testosterone receptors in human benign and malignant prostatic tumors

2.9.2.1. pH effect

One hundred microliters (350 μg protein) of purified receptors were completed to 0.5 ml with distilled water at different pH (2,6,7.2,8.2,9.2,and 12) then each of which was placed in the test cell and the adjusted pH distilled water was placed in the reference cell and the absorption spectra of different purified receptors were measured immediately.

2.9.2.2. Polarity effect

a. The effect of 20% ethanol on the testosterone receptors spectra:

One hundred microliters (350 μg protein) of purified receptors were completed to 0.5 ml with distilled water contains 20% ethanol at pH 7.2 then each of which was placed in the test cell and the 20% ethanol adjusted pH was placed in the reference cell using 0.5 cm cuvette. The absorption spectrum of each sample was measured immediately.

b. The effect of 20% ethylene glycol on the testosterone receptors spectra:

One hundred microliters (350 μg protein) of purified receptors were completed to 0.5 ml with distilled water contains 20% ethylene glycol at pH 7.2 then each of which was placed in the test cell and the 20% ethylene glycol adjusted pH was placed in the reference cell using 0.5 cm cuvette. The absorption spectrum of each sample was measured immediately.

c. The effect of 20% urea on the testosterone receptors spectra:

One hundred microliters (350 μg protein) of purified nuclear receptors were completed to 0.5 ml with distilled water at pH 7.2 containing 20% urea then placed in the test cell against the 20% urea adjusted pH in the reference cell using 0.5 cm cuvette. The absorption spectra of different purified receptors were measured immediately.

d. The effect of NaCl and CaCl₂ on the testosterone receptors spectra:

One hundred microliters (350 µg protein) of purified nuclear receptors were completed to 0.5 ml with distilled water at pH 7.2 containing separately 0.1 M NaCl and 25 mM CaCl₂, then each of which was placed in a 0.5 cm cuvette in the test beam against an appropriate blank in the reference beam. The absorption spectra were measured immediately.

Solutions

- 25 mM CaCl₂ solution was prepared by dissolving 0.2774 gm of CaCl₂ in 100 ml distilled water. The pH required was then adjusted.
- 0.1 M NaCl soultion was prepared by dissolving 0.5844 gm of NaCl in 100 ml distilled water. The pH required was then adjusted.

2.9.3. The effect of 10% cisplatin drug on the testosterone receptors spectra

One hundred microliters (350 µg protein) of purified receptors were completed to 0.5 ml with distilled water at pH 7.2 containing 10% cisplatin drug, then placed in the test cell against the 10% cisplatin adjusted pHsolution in the reference cell using 0.5 cm cuvette. The absorption spectra of different purified receptors were measured immediately.

2.9.4. Spectrophotometric pH titration of purified nuclear testosterone receptors in human benign and malignant prostatic tumors

A series of purified nuclear receptors (350 µg protein in 100 µl) were completed to 0.5 ml with distilled water at pH ranging from 9.0 to 12.5. The maximum absorbance of each sample was measured at a wavelength of 295 nm, the absorbance of λ_{max} at each pH value was plotted versus the corresponding pH.

Another series of purified receptors were completed to 0.5 ml with distilled water at pH range from 4 to 8.0. The maximum absorbance of each sample was measured at a wavelength of 211 nm. The absorbance of λ_{max} at each pH value was plotted against the corresponding pH.

2.9.5. Observation of the helix coil transition of the purified nuclear testosterone receptors of human benign and malignant prostatic tumors

One hundred microliters (350 µg protein) of purified nuclear receptors were completed to 0.5 ml with 20% ethylene glycol and 0.01 M NaCl dissolved in distilled water at pH 7.2. Each mixture was placed in 0.5 cm cuvette in the sample beam and the maximum absorbance of each purified receptor was measured at a wavelength of 292 nm at increasing temperatures (20 to 70°C) against the reference (ethylene glycol-NaCl adjusted pH solution).

The maximum absorbance of each purified receptor was plotted against the different temperatures. The experiment was repeated for each purified receptor with another solution (20% ethylene glycol-0.1M NaCl).

2.9.6. The U.V. spectra of ^{125}I-testosterone and the different ^{125}I-testosterone receptor complexes

2.9.6.1. The U.V. spectra of different human testosterone-receptors complexes of benign and malignant prostatic tumors

The binding experiment of different purified nuclear testosterone receptors with ^{125}I-testosterone was carried out at the optimum conditions as explained previously in sections (2.8.1) and (2.8.2). Half milliliter of the ^{125}I-testosterone-receptor complex supernatant of each type of purified receptors was placed in 0.5cm cuvette in the sample beam and the absorption spectrum was measured immediately against an appropriate blank in the reference beam.

2.9.6.2. The U.V-spectrum of ^{125}I-testosterone

Half milliliter of ^{125}I-testosterone was placed in a 0.5cm cuvette in the sample beam and the absorption spectrum was measured immediately against an appropriate blank in the reference beam.

2.10. Statistical analysis

The results of serum testosterone, iron, copper, zinc, calcium, magnesium, copper/zinc ratio and magnesium/calcium ratio were analyzed statistically and values were expressed as mean ± SD. The levels of significance were determined by student's t-test [53].

CHAPTER 3

Results & Discussion

Results and Discussion

3.1. Evaluation of some biochemical constituents in sera and tissues of prostatic tumors patients

3.1.1. Determination of testosterone levels in sera of prostatic tumors patients

Testosterone levels in sera of patients with BPH (group I) and PCA (group II) were measured by radioimmuno assay [116,117]. The two groups were matched with a group of control subjects.

Table (3-1) shows the results obtained from this study. The level of serum testosterone in BPH patients was found to be 4 ng/ml, whereas that of PCA patients was found to be 3.923 ng/ml. But in controls, the level was found to be 4.33 ng/ml. Student's t-test analysis revealed that the means of the groups were significantly non different ($p < 0.1$).

Table (3-1): Serum testosterone levels (ng/ml) in patients with BPH and PCA. Details are described in section (2.2.1).

Group	No. of cases	Age (year)	Serum testosterone (ng/ml)
I (BPH)	25	65.95±1.15	4 ± 0.655
II (PCA)	3	73.66±0.62	3.923 ± 1.024
Control	16	68±1.9	4.33 ± 0.20

These results are nearly similar to those obtained previously by other investigators [118,119,135], Habib et al reported that there were no significant differences between the peripheral plasma concentrations of testosterone in BPH and in carcinoma, also reported that the testosterone level in patients affected with BPH was 5.6 ± 0.7 ng/ml while in patients with PCA was 4.8 ± 0.8 ng/ml [119].

Eriksson and Carlström (1988) underlined that the plasma testosterone may be in normal level or slightlydecreasedin PCA [118].

3.1.2. Determination of testosterone levels in human benign and malignant prostatic tissues

Testosterone was measured in the crude nuclear fraction of benign and malignant prostatic tissues. The level in BPH tissues was found to be significantly different from that of the level in PCA tissues. The concentration in benign tumor tissues was found to be 6.32 μg/g of tissue while in malignant tumor tissue the concentration was 5.6 μg/g of tissue.

These results indicated that there was a decrease in testosterone level in malignant prostatic tumor tissue compared with that of benign prostatic tumors tissue, this finding may be attributed to an elevated activities of 5α-reductase in malignant prostatic tumors compared with those of benign tumors and normal prostates [11,13,119-125].

3.1.3. Determination of iron, copper, zinc, calcium and magnesium in sera of patients with benign and malignant prostatic tumors

Iron, copper, zinc, calcium and magnesium were measured in sera of patients with benign and malignant prostatic tumors by atomic absorption spectrophotometry [103-105].

Many disease states, including hepatic disease affect plasma trace elements, i.e., iron, copper and zinc levels [126]. Hence patients with such diseases were excluded from this study. The mean serum concentrations of these elements ± SD are shown in Table (3-2). The results showed that serum iron levels were very significantly higher ($P < 0.0005$) in benign prostatic tumor patients than those in the control group, while remained with small significant increase ($P < 0.1$) in the group of malignant tumor patients. Serum copper levels were very significantly increased($P < 0.00025$) in benign prostatic tumor patients than those in control group, while very high significant increase ($P < 0.001$) in the group of malignant tumor patients. Serum zinc levels elevated significantly ($P < 0.1$) in sera of patients with benign tumors and decreased high significantly ($P < 0.01$) in sera of patients with malignant tumors when compared with normal individuals. On the other hand, serum calcium levels were very significantly ($P < 0.001$) lower in sera of benign tumors but not in patients with malignant tumors ($P < 0.1$) when compared with those of controls. Finally it was found that serum magnesium levels were increased very high significantly ($P < 0.00001$) in benign tumor patients and ($P < 0.0025$) in malignant tumor patients when compared with those of controls. The most important finding was the usefulness of the ratios of copper to zinc and magnesium to calcium. They were increased very highly significant ($P < 0.00001$) in malignant tumor patients than those of controls, also in benign tumors the increase in both ratios were very highly significant ($P < 0.0001$ for Cu/Zn ratio and $P < 0.00001$ for Mg/Ca ratio). The increase of Cu/Zn ratio in sera of prostatic adenocarcinoma patients reflects the implication of the two elements, i.e., copper and zinc in the cancerous process of the prostatic tissues, so this ratio as well as the Mg/Ca ratio may be used as a biochemical marker for the evaluation of the status of prostate cancer patients, discrimination between benign and malignant tumor patients and also could be used as one of the parameters reflecting the outcome of therapy. Decreased levels of zinc with increased levels of copper are found in sera of malignant prostatic tumor patients. In addition, the levels of iron were increased significantly ($P < 0.1$). These results may indicate the presence of interrelationships between copper, iron and zinc in the initiation and growth of malignant prostatic tumors. The zinc levels are usually low and copper levels are high in the plasma of most cancer patients [127,128]. However, the results obtained in this study reflect this. It has been postulated that the lowering of plasma zinc is due to a shift of the element from the transport medium to the liver as a protective mechanism against the spread of cancer. It was possible that prostatic tumor tissue, which requires high concentration of zinc for its proliferation, may have developed techniques for extracting zinc from the circulation [104,129-131]. The explanation of the depression of zinc levels in sera of patients with prostate cancer may be attributed to the increase in the testosterone receptor synthesis rate, this process increases the zinc uptake from the circulation to incorporate it at the zinc fingers of the DNA-binding domain in the testosterone receptor, each receptor molecule synthesized consumes two zinc atoms [74,75], or in another simple word testosterone hormone action is a zinc dependent process, so, these receptors require zinc to bind to the genes they activate, in cancer these processes (testosterone receptor synthesis and action) were accelerated and thereby increasing the consumption of zinc from the circulation [105].

When zinc levels are low in plasma, there are more binding sites in the albumin for non-specific transport of copper. The high concentration of copper found in the plasma of patients with a number of disorders including cancer, is bound to albumin [130]. The exact mechanism by which copper concentrations are increased during cancer are not well understood at present.

From these results it was found that prostate cancer patients have lower values of calcium concentrations compared with normal individuals in contrast to that obtained previously for other types of cancers [55,103,132].

Table (3-2): Iron, copper, zinc, calcium and magnesium levels in sera of patients with benign and malignant prostatic tumors and in age matched healthy individuals as a control. All details are explained in section (2.2.3).

Element	BPH	PCA	Control
Fe (ppm)	3.594± 0.746	2.546± 1.011	1.78± 0.347
Cu (ppm)	2.017± 0.372	1.72± 0.113	0.882± 0.214
Zn (ppm)	1.428± 0.363	0.7± 0.07	1.108± 0.198
Ca (ppm)	67.743± 4.041	75.9± 5.303	80.45± 2.174
Mg (ppm)	23.485± 0.293	29.4± 2.97	18.266± 1.03
Cu/Zn	1.704± 0.278	2.475± 0.083	0.8611± 0.173
Mg/Ca	0.353± 0.021	0.385± 0.011	0.227± 0.015

3.2. Binding studies of ^{125}I-testosterone with its crude receptors in human benign and malignant prostatic tumors

2.2.1. Preliminary test of ^{125}I-testosterone binding to its crude nuclear receptors in prostatic tumors homogenates

By using prostatic tumor homogenate as the source of testosterone receptors, cytosolic and nuclear receptors were investigated in benign and malignant prostatic tumors. According to the radioreceptor technique, there were no detectable levels of cytosolic testosterone receptors in human benign and malignant prostatic tumors. The lack of these receptors may be explained by intranuclear accumulation of testosterone receptor complexes [38, 156].

Nuclear testosterone receptors were detected through the incubation of ^{125}I-testosterone with crude nuclear fraction and the bound testosterone was separated by dextran-coated charcoal method and then measured by γ-counter. The specific binding was found to be 6% in benign prostatic tumors and 3% in prostatic adenocarcinoma tumors. The data obtained in this preliminary experiment revealed the presence of nuclear testosterone receptors in human benign and malignant prostatic tumors.

3.2.2. Factors affecting the binding of ^{125}I-testosterone to its crude benign and malignant prostatic tumors receptors

3.2.2.1. The effect of different concentrations of testosterone receptors (DNA or protein) on the binding of ^{125}I-testosterone in prostatic tumor homogenate

In order to demonstrate whether the specific binding was proportional to the amount of testosterone receptors (DNA or proteins) used, increasing amounts of nuclear homogenate were incubated with ^{125}I-testosterone with and without the addition of nonradioactive testosterone, according to the details in section (2.4.1). As shown in Figure (3-1A &B), the specific binding percent was increased when the amount of receptor protein in the incubation mixture was increased. In all the subsequent experiments, 200 μg of receptor protein (or 360 μg DNA) of benign crude nuclear homogenate and 150 μg of receptor protein (or 450 μg DNA) of malignant crude nuclear homogenate were used.

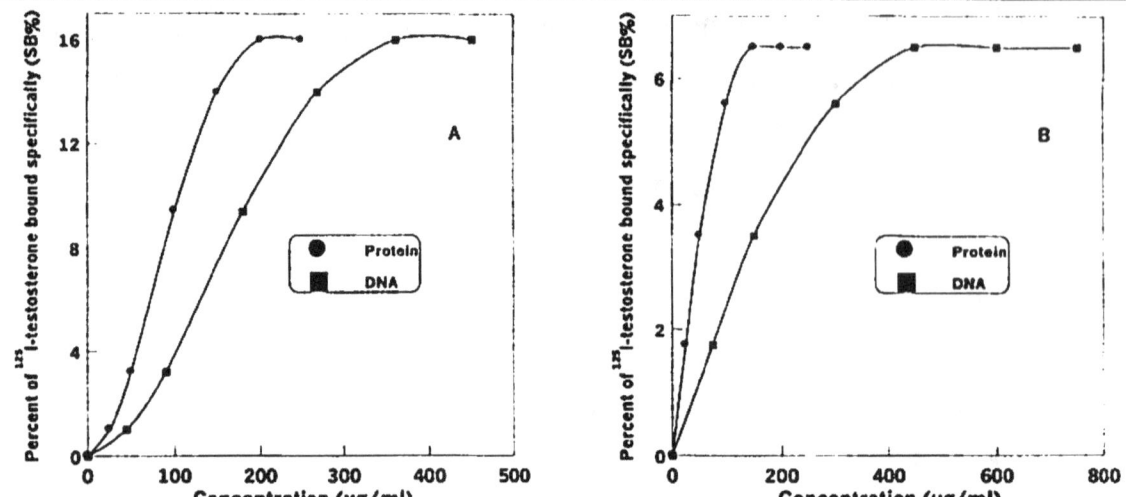

Figure (3-1): Influence of crude testosterone receptor concentration (protein and DNA) on the binding of ^{125}I-testosterone with: A) Benign prostatic tumor homogenate, B) Malignant prostatic tumor homogenate. Details are described in section (2.4.1).

3.2.2.2. The effect of different concentrations of ^{125}I-testosterone on the binding with its crude nuclear receptors in benign and malignant prostatic tumors

One of the most important criteria of the hormone receptors is its saturability. To fulfil this criterion and to estimate the suitable concentration of ^{125}I-testosterone, the experiment was carried out as mentioned previously in section (2.4.2). The results revealed that the testosterone binding by nuclear fractions is a saturable process and as shown in the Figure (3-2), the nuclear receptor protein used in the incubation mixtures under the conditions of the experiment were saturated (8.7 PM of ^{125}I-testosterone for benign nuclear receptors) and (4.35 PM of ^{125}I-testosterone for malignant nuclear receptors). Accordingly, in all the subsequent experiments, the above concentrations of ^{125}I-testosterone were used.

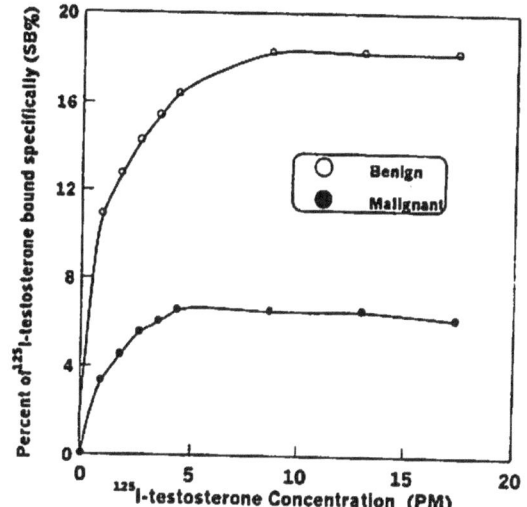

Figure (3-2): Effect of different concentrations of ¹²⁵I-testosterone on the binding with its prostatic receptors. Details are described in section (2.4.2).

3.2.2.3. *Effect of pH on the binding of ¹²⁵I-testosterone to its receptors in benign and malignant prostatic tumors*

The effect of pH on the specific binding of ^{125}I-testosterone to its receptors was investigated. Figure (3-3) shows that the optimum pH was found to be 7.8 for the binding of benign receptors and 8.5 for the binding of malignant receptors. The dissociation of testosterone–receptor complex occurs greatly at pH 7.2 and 9.0, also these results indicate that the binding was pH-dependent and the shift in the pH of the environment may affect the properties of the macromolecules involved in the binding. This effect includes the induction of protonation-deprotonation processes occurring with the ionizable groups of the amino acids present in the binding domain of these macromolecules [133]. In view of these results, the buffers in all subsequent experiments were adjusted to pH 7.8 for benign tumors and pH 8.5 for malignant tumors.

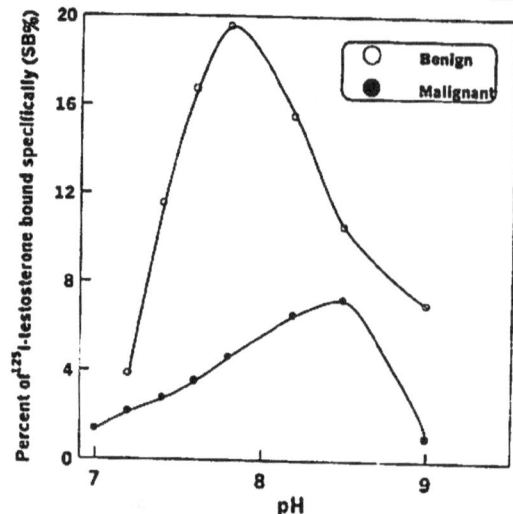

Figure (3–3): pH dependency of ^{125}I-testosterone binding with its prostatic receptors. All details are described in section (2.4.3).

3.2.2.4. The choice of most appropriate incubation time of ^{125}I-testosterone binding to its receptors in prostatic tumor homogenate

The time course of the binding of testosterone to its receptors was investigated by incubating nuclear fractions of benign and malignant prostatic tumors for the time indicated at 4°C with and without the addition of unlabeled testosterone. Figure (3-4) shows that the specific binding of ^{125}I-testosterone to its receptors was maximal at 16 h for benign and malignant tumors.

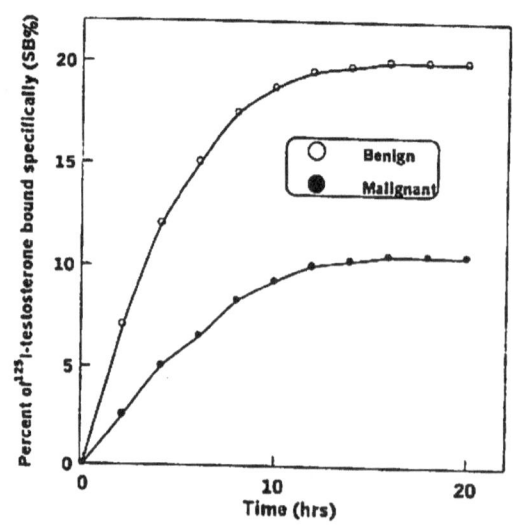

Figure (3–4): Time course of ^{125}I-testosterone binding with its prostatic receptors. All details are described in section (2.4.4).

3.2.2.5. Temperature dependency of the binding between ^{125}I-testosterone and their receptors in benign and malignant prostatic tumors

Temperature dependency of the association of ^{125}I-testosterone to its nuclear receptors was investigated. Nuclear fractions of benign and malignant prostatic tumors were incubated for 16 hrs at different temperatures (4-55°C). Figure (3-5) revealed that the specific binding of ^{125}I-testosterone to its nuclear receptors was increased when the temperature was raised from 4 to 37°C for benign tumors and from 4 to 45°C for malignant tumors. The loss of binding activity may be due to denaturation of receptor molecules or to the irreversible dissociation of testosterone-receptor complex. According to the results of this experiment, the binding studies of the subsequent investigations were carried out with 16 hrs at 37°C for benign receptors and at 45°C for malignant receptors. These results are nearly similar to that obtained by King and Mainwaring who found that most steroid receptors are irreversibly destroyed above 45°C [134].

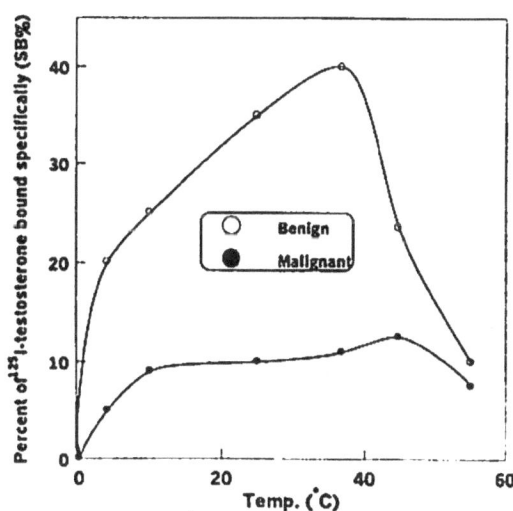

Figure (3-5): Effect of temperature on ^{125}I-testosterone binding with its prostatic receptors. All details are described in section (2.4.5).

3.2.2.6. The effect of different halides on the binding of ^{125}I-testosterone to its receptors

Figure (3-6) shows the effect of different halide salts (i.e., NaF, NaCl and NaI) at 0.1 M concentration on the extent of ^{125}I-testosterone binding to their receptors in benign and malignant prostatic tumors   .The sodium halides in the incubation mixture of benign and malignant receptors induced activation of the percent of specific binding according to the following sequence:

$$NaF < NaCl < NaI$$

Melander and Horvath (1977) reported that the effect of halide salt type on hydrophobic interactions is quantified by its molal surface tension increment (MSTI) which is a measure of the increase in surface tension by the salt, also they found that this parameter increases as the following sequence:

$$NaF > NaCl > NaI$$

The same researchers found that halides with higher MSTI values will strengthen the hydrophobic interactions while halides with lower MSTI values reverse this effect. Thus the dependence of the extent of specific binding of ^{125}I-testosterone with its receptors in benign and malignant tumors on MSTI value of the corresponding halide further implicates the low involvement of hydrophobic forces in maintaining the stability of ^{125}I-testosterone-receptor complexes formed[(136)].

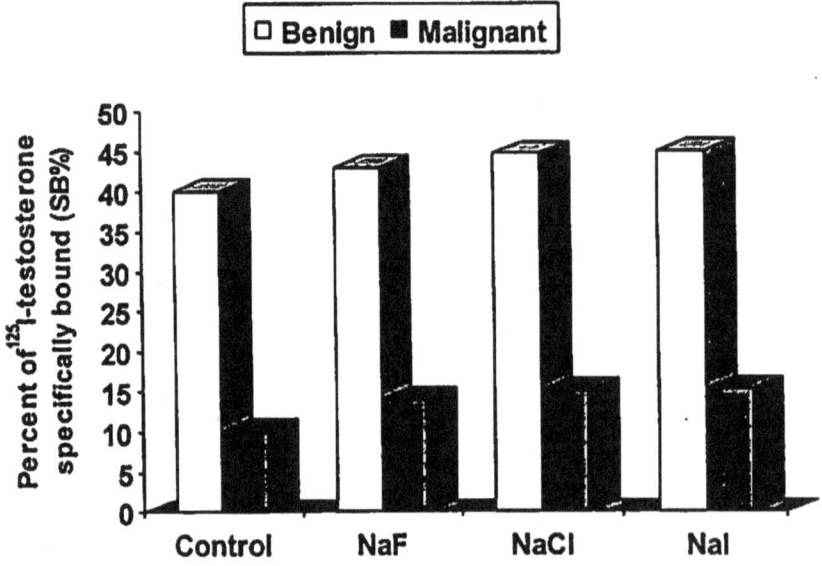

Figure (3–6): Effect of different halides on the extent of
[125]I-testosterone binding with its prostatic receptors. All
details are described in section (2.4.6).

3.2.2.7. The effect of monovalent and divalent salts on the binding of ^{125}I-testosterone to its nuclear receptors in benign and malignant prostatic tumors

Figure (3-7) shows the effect of different salts on the extent of the binding of ^{125}I-testosterone to its receptors in benign and malignant prostatic tumors. $CaCl_2$ at 25 mM was shown to increase the binding by more than 20% of the control value in benign tumors while $MgCl_2$ at the same concentration activated the binding to more than 91% of the control value in malignant tumors. The other salts ($NaCl$, NH_4Cl, $CsCl$, KCl, $LiCl$, $CuSO_4.5H_2O$ and $MnCl_2.4H_2O$) also increased the binding but to a lesser extent.

From the results illustrated in Figure (3-7), it is suggested that these salts may provide some conformational changes in the testosterone receptors and the charged groups of the binding domain of these receptors that hinder maximal binding are shielded [65,137,138].

Among all cations studied the calcium ion was the most important for the stimulation of testosterone binding to its prostatic receptors, these results may suggest that testosterone binding is a calmoduline dependent process [139].

The inhibiting effect of Zn(II) ions on the testosterone binding to its receptors in these results are in agreement with those of other authors who found in their experiments that zinc was capable of binding with specific sites on steroid receptor molecule and then inhibiting the steroid binding [129,131,138].

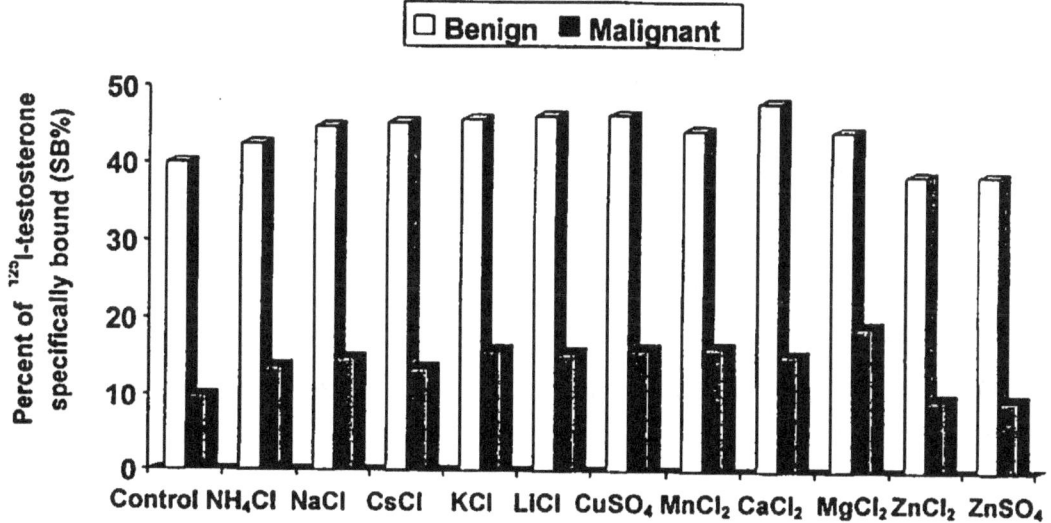

Figure (3-7): Effects of monovalent and divalent cations on the binding of ^{125}I-testosterone with its prostatic receptors. All details are described in sections (2.4.7) and (2.4.8).

3.2.2.8. The choice of most appropriate concentration of β-mercaptoethanol for the binding of ^{125}I-testosterone with their receptors

The inclusion of thiol reagents such as β-mercaptoethanol helps to stabilize steroid receptor proteins [134] and to protect protein thiols from oxidation [101]. From this experiment it was found that the most appropriate concentration of β-mercaptoethanol was 2.5 mM in benign tumors with an activation percent of 10% of control value and 10 mM in malignant tumors with an activation percent of 50% of control value.

These results are shown in Figure (3-8).

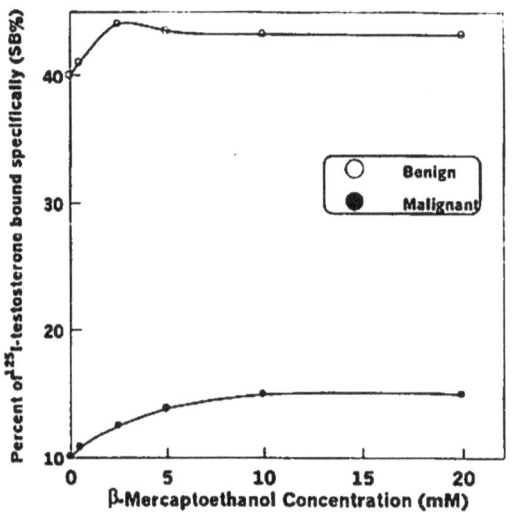

Figure (3–8): Effect of β-mercaptoethanol on the binding of ^{125}I-testosterone with its prostatic receptors. All details are described in section (2.4.9).

The marked increase in specific binding of ^{125}I-testosterone to its benign and malignant prostatic tumor receptors with increasing thiol reagent concentration may indicate the presence of sulfhydryl groups (-SH) which may be located either at the testosterone binding site of the receptor or at some distal site whose integrity is essential to the proper conformation of the testosterone binding domain [140-142].

3.2.2.9. The effect of urea on the binding of ¹²⁵I-testosterone with its receptors

Figure (3-9) shows the effect of different concentrations of urea on the specific binding of ¹²⁵I-testosterone to its receptors. These experimental results showed that the addition of urea (concentrations ranging from 0.1 M to 4 M) resulted in a gradual dissociation of the complex. The urea at 4 M was able to dissociate about 12.5% of benign complexes and about 25% of malignant complexes, this may be attributed to the effect of urea on the hydrophobic forces participitating in the association of protein molecules [143].

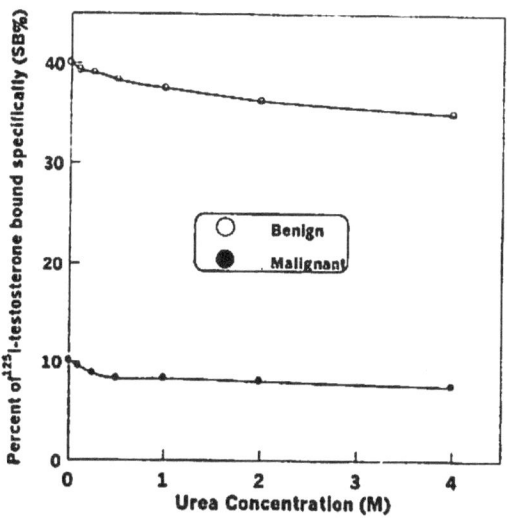

Figure (3–9): Effect of different urea concentrations on the binding of ¹²⁵I-testosterone with its prostatic receptors. All details are described in section (2.4.10).

3.2.2.10. The effect of polyethylene glycol (PEG-6000) on the binding of ¹²⁵I-testosterone to its benign and malignant prostatic tumors receptors

Figure (3-10) shows the effect of different concentrations of PEG-6000 on the specific binding of ¹²⁵I-testosterone to its receptors. The experimental results showed that addition of PEG ranging in concentration from (1 to 6%) resulted in a gradual decrease of specific binding percent. Therefore, it was found that 6% of this polymer causes more than 31% precipitation of benign receptors and about 20% of malignant receptors. The effect of PEG on the receptor protein solubility can be explained according to the steric exclusion mechanism proposed by

Laurent [144], assuming a fixed total volume (V_T) of solvent being occupied by both polymer and protein, and defining the volume occupied by polymer as (V_E) (excluded volume i.e., volume not accessible to proteins) and the volume occupied by protein as (V'). The relation ($V_T = V' + V_E$) implies that any increase in V_E, due to increase in number or size of polymer molecules, forces a decrease in (V') and an effective increase in the concentration of protein molecules. Hence, as V_E is increased, the effective protein concentration increased as well as collision and self association of protein molecules thereby enhancing the protein precipitation because of the formation of large insoluble aggregates [144,101].

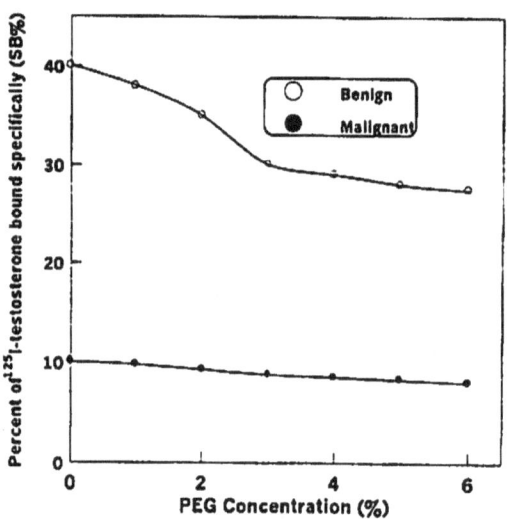

Figure (3–10): Effect of different concentrations of PEG 6000 on the resulted specific binding of ^{125}I-testosterone with its prostatic receptors. All details are described in section (2.4.11).

3.2.2.11. The effect of molybdate ion on the binding of ^{125}I-testosterone to its receptors in benign and malignant prostatic tumors

The stabilizing effects of molybdate ion on steroid receptors have been described by many investigators [140,145-149].

Thompson and Chung (1984) in their study on rat prostate suggested that molybdate not only interacts directly with cytosolic androgen receptors but also interacts with particulate fractions of the homogenate such as the prostatic nuclei to form relatively more stable complex [145].

In this study it was found that the binding in the presence of moybdate, as shown in Figure (3-11), is approximately 12% higher than in its absence at the most appropriate concentration (1.5 mM) for benign receptors and more than 36% higher than the control value at the most appropriate concentration (0.5 mM) for malignant receptors. These results are in consistent with those reported previously[140,146-149].

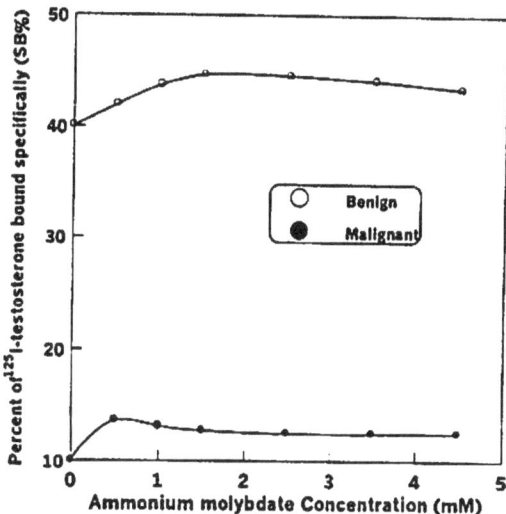

Figure (3–11): Effect of different concentrations of molybdate ion on the resulted specific binding of ^{125}**I-testosterone with its prostatic receptors. All details are described in section (2.4.12).**

3.2.2.12. The effect of N-bromosuccinimide (NBS) on the binding of ^{125}I-testosterone with its receptors in benign and malignant prostatic tumors

Figure (3-12) shows that the incubation of ^{125}I-testosterone with its benign and malignant prostatic tumors receptors in the presence of NBS ranging in concentration from (5 to 40 mM) resulted in a gradual dissociation of the testosterone-receptors complexes. NBS at 40 mM concentration was shown to dissociate more than 62% of benign testosterone-receptor complexes formed and 30% of the malignant testosterone-receptor complexes formed.

Many investigators reported that NBS has specificity toward tryptophan and cystein residues. Thus the inhibition of binding in the presence of NBS suggests that both tryptophan and cystein residues are necessary for maintaining the functional configuration of the binding active site and the stability of the complex formed [65,142,150,151].

The results in this study are in consistent with those reported previously that testosterone receptor active site at different species contains tryptophan residues[134,142,152].

From our results, it was concluded that benign receptor active site contains more tryptophan and cystein residues number than the malignant receptor active site.

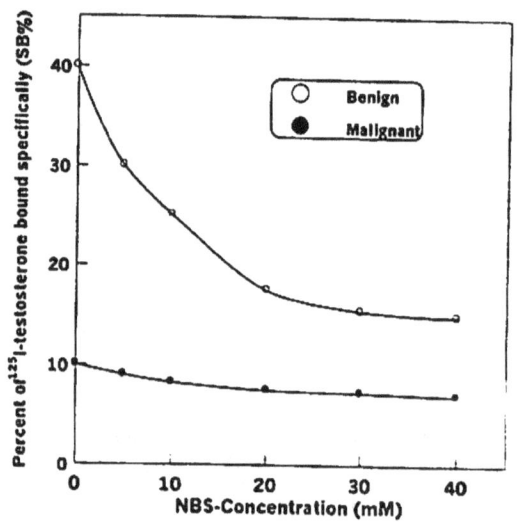

Figure (3–12): Effect of different concentrations of NBS on the resulted specific binding of ^{125}I-testosterone with its benign and malignant prostatic receptors. All details are described in section (2.4.13).

3.2.2.13. Stability of ^{125}I-testosterone-receptors complexes of benign and malignant prostatic tumors

The influence of temperature on the stability of testosterone-receptor complex as a function of time was studied. The complexes of benign and malignant prostatic receptors were reincubated at four temperatures (0,4,10,25°C) and at certain time intervals the remaining bound testosterone was estimated. As seen in Figure (3-13A&B), the rate of dissociation of testosterone-nuclear receptor complex was increased as the temperature increased leading to an almost complete elimination of specific binding at 25°C after 90 min for benign receptor complexes and to about 89% dissociation of the malignant receptor complexes. The dissociation at 0°C of both testosterone-receptors complexes is very weak.

The results of this experiment stated clearly that the malignant receptor was more thermostable than the benign receptor and the temperature sensitivity of testosterone-receptor complexes was at temperature more than 4°C. Thus our results are nearly similar to that obtained by King and Mainwaring who they found that most steroid receptors are irreversibly destroyed above 45°C [134].

Other investigators showed that the heating of cytosolic human androgen receptor at 50°C for 30 min destroyed more than 72% of receptor complexes and the incubation of the complex for 16 hr at 4°C resulted in a 46% decrease in the androgen-receptor complex formation [153].

A group of scientists underlined that the complex was stable at 0°C for at least 20 hr [154] while another group showed that the complex is stable at 0°C for long periods but it is rapidly degraded at temperatures of 37°C and above [65].

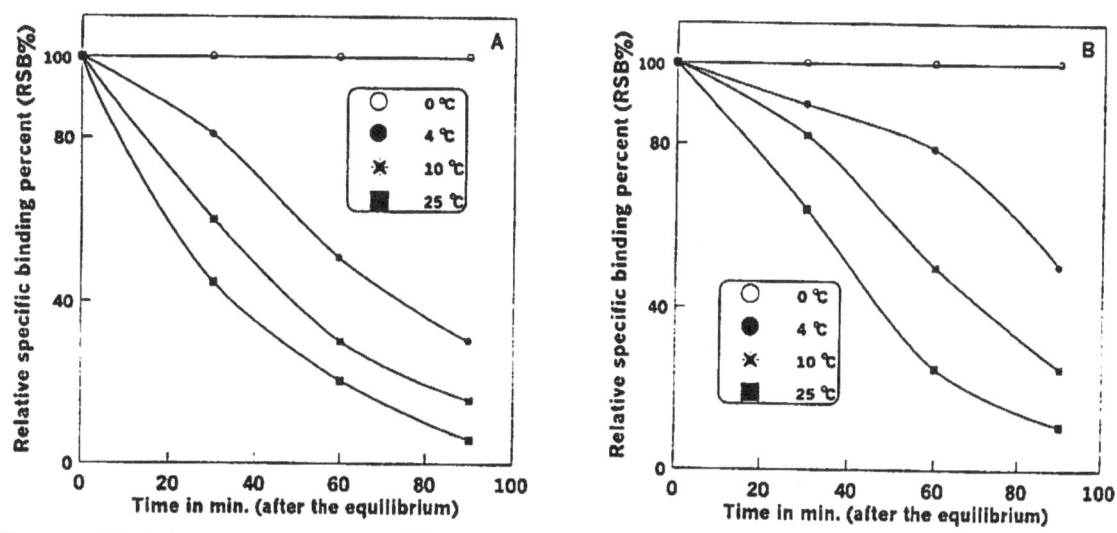

Figure (3–13): Stability of ¹²⁵I-testosterone-receptor complex of, A) benign prostatic tumor homogenate, b) malignant prostatic tumor homogenate at four different temperatures. All details are described in section (2.4.14).

3.2.2.14. Competitive effect of different concentrations of unlabeled testosterone, estrone and estriol on the binding of ¹²⁵I-testosterone to its receptors in human benign and malignant prostatic tumors

The specificity of benign and malignant testosterone receptors for binding with different steroids were demonstrated by a decrease in receptor bound radioactivity after incubating the nuclear fraction with increasing amounts of unlabeled steroid hormones. Figure (3-14A) shows that the binding of ¹²⁵I-testosterone to its benign receptors was effectively inhibited by unlabeled testosterone and with a lesser extent by unlabeled estriol while 500 nM of unlabeled estrone causes only 10% loss of ^{125}I-testosterone binding. Different pattern of inhibition was observed in Figure (3-14B) for malignant receptors. The frequency of inhibiting strength of these steroids was found to be as the following:

Estriol > Estrone > Testosterone

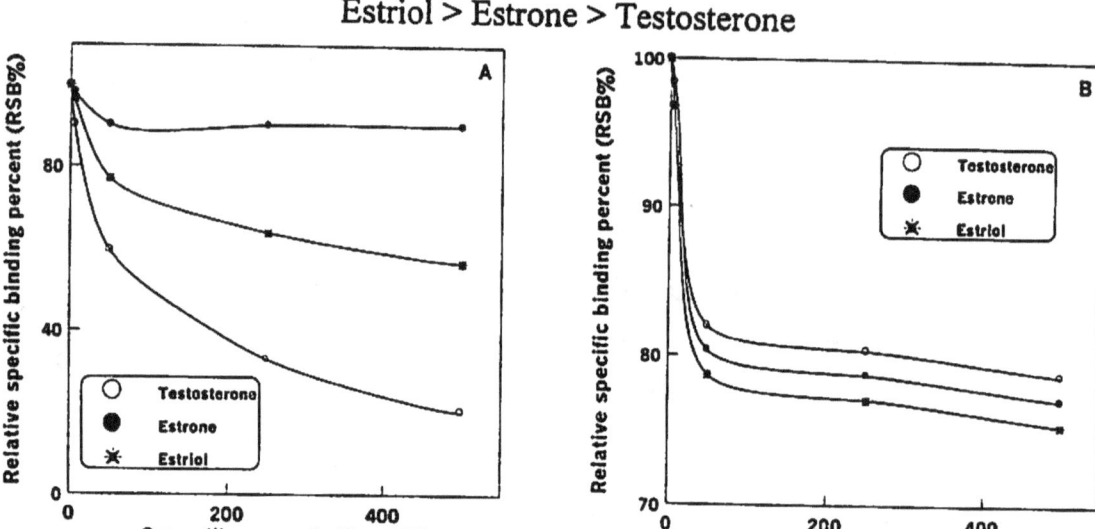

Figure (3-14): Binding of, A) benign prostatic nuclear receptors, B) malignant prostatic nuclear receptors with ^{125}I-testosterone in the presence of different concentrations of unlabeled competitors . All details are described in section (2.4.15).

The difference in inhibition patterns between benign and malignant nuclear receptors may be attributed to the structural differences of the two types of receptors. The competition index values were calculated from the relative competition plot in Figure (3-15 A&B) and the values obtained were summarized in Table (3-3).

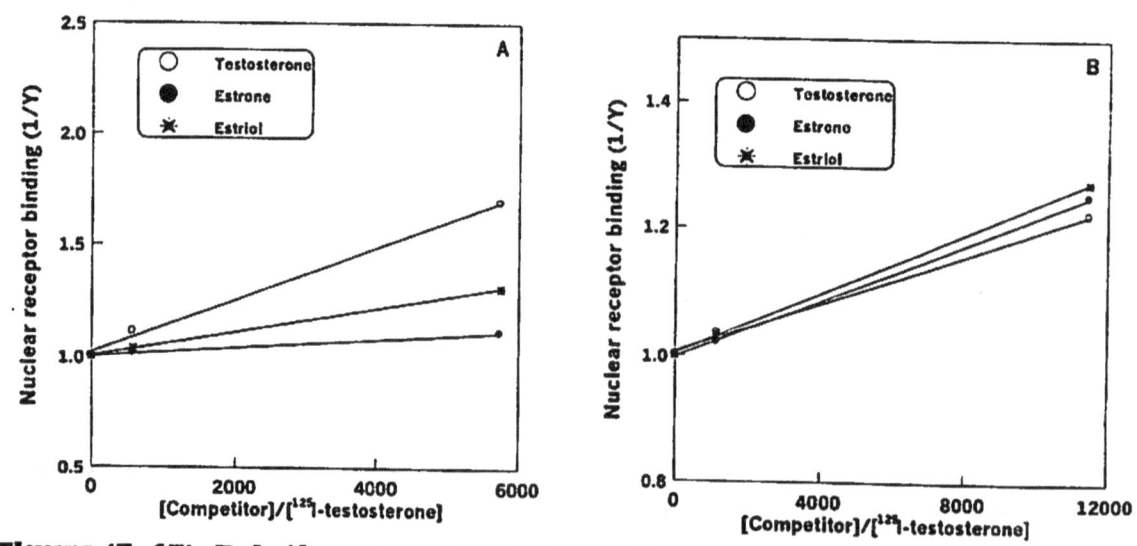

Figure (3-15): Relative competition (RC) plot of increasing concentrations of unlabeled competing steroids with ^{125}I-testosterone for the binding with its A) benign, B) malignant, prostatic receptors. All details are described in section (2.4.15).

Relative competition index (RCI) values of benign and malignant nuclear receptors for different unlabeled steroids were obtained as described previously in section (2.4.15) and summarized in Table (3-4).

Table (3-3): Competition index values (a) for different steroids competing with ^{125}I-testosterone for binding with benign and malignant prostatic tumors receptors. Details are described in section (2.4.15).

Competitor	Competition index (a) for benign receptors ($\times 10^{-3}$)	Competition index (a) for malignant receptors ($\times 10^{-3}$)
Testosterone	0.116	0.020
Estrone	0.020	0.021
Estriol	0.057	0.025

Table (3-4): Relative competition index values (RCI) for different steroids competing with ^{125}I-testosterone for binding with benign and malignant prostatic tumors receptors. Details are described in section (2.4.15).

Competitor	Relative Competition index (RCI) for benign receptors	Relative competition index (RCI) for malignant receptors
Testosterone	1.0	1.0
Estrone	0.172	1.055
Estriol	0.492	1.250

These results indicated that testosterone binds to nuclear androgen receptor in human prostate with high specificity compared with the other competitors. Our results are in agreement with the results of many authors stated previously[102,108,154,155].

3.3. The kinetics and thermodynamics of the interaction of testosterone with its crude nuclear receptors

3.3.1. Kinetics of the ^{125}I-testosterone binding to its crude receptors in benign and malignant prostatic tumors

Figure (3-16 A&B) shows the time course of the formation of ^{125}I-testosterone-receptor complex at five different temperatures (4,10,25,37 and 45°C) in benign and malignant prostatic tumors. The results of time course patterns at different temperatures revealed that the binding of ^{125}I-testosterone to its receptors in prostatic tumors is a temperature and time dependent process with a maximum binding occurs at 37°C with 16 hr for benign receptors and at 45°C with 16 hr for malignant receptors.

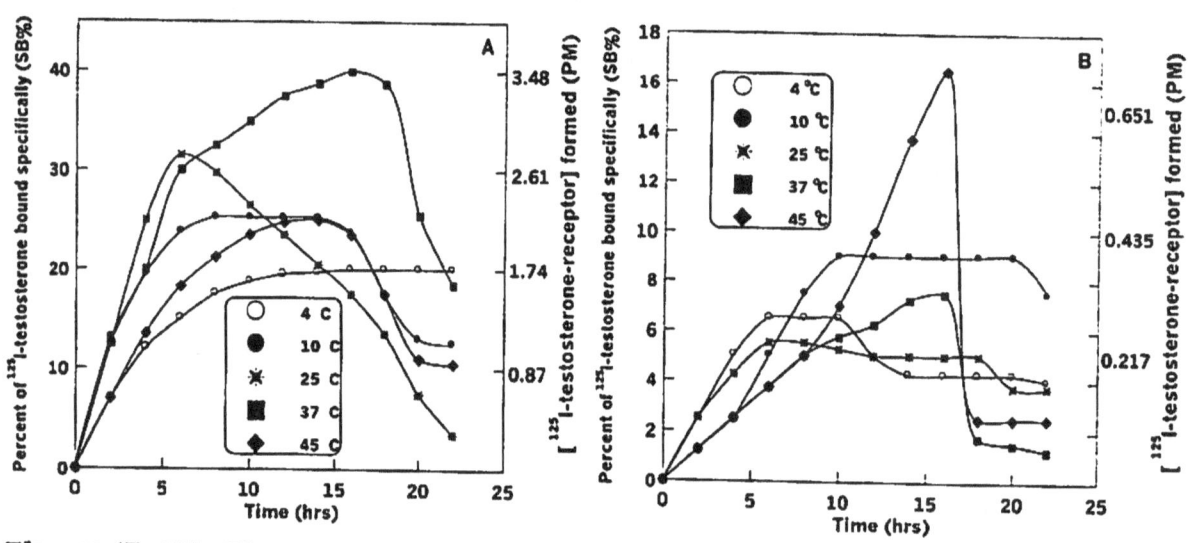

Figure (3–16): Time course of the association of ^{125}I-testosterone with its, A) benign prostatic receptors, B) malignant prostatic receptors at different temperatures. All details are described in section (2.5.1).

3.3.1.1. *Determination of the concentrations and affinity constants of testosterone receptors in human benign and malignant prostatic tumors*

Nuclear testosterone receptor concentrations and the affinity constants have been measured in benign and malignant prostatic tumors. The experiment was carried out at the optimal conditions, which were obtained in previous experiments and was repeated at different temperatures (4,10,25,37 and 45°C). Scatchard plot analysis gave a straight line as shown in Figure (3-17 A&B) at each temperature indicating the presence of only one species of receptor site, or more but with the same affinity and number of binding sites.

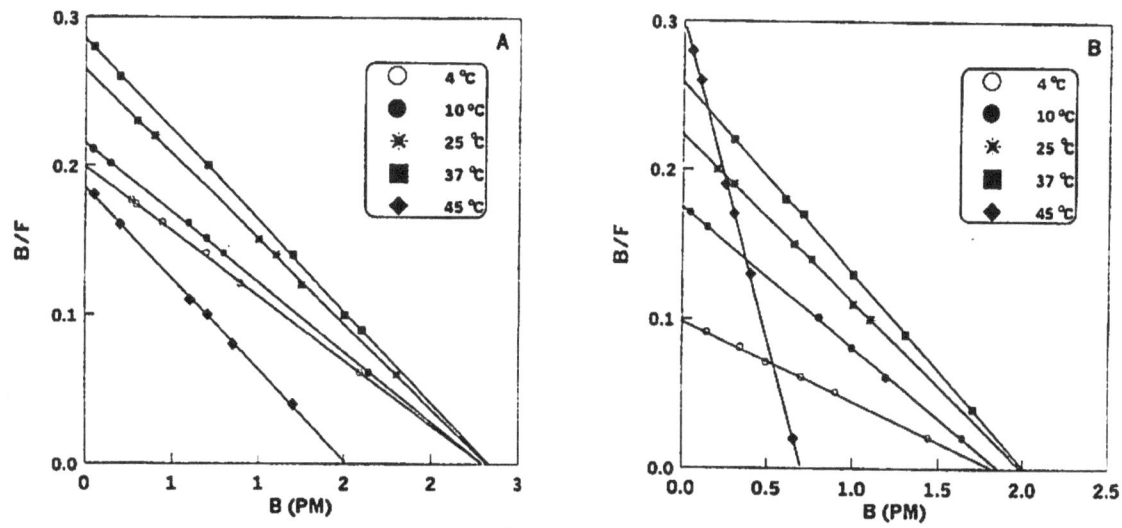

Figure (3–17): Scatchard plot of ^{125}I-testosterone binding with its, A) benign prostatic receptors, B) malignant prostatic receptors at five different temperatures. All details are described in section (2.5.2).

The results are summarized in Table (3-5). Testosterone receptor measurements in prostatic carcinoma may help the clinician to select the optimal therapy (endocrine versus non-endocrine) in the individual case and also possibly to select the more appropriate form of endocrine treatment. Patients with "receptor-rich" tumors might be considered for alternative forms of hormonal treatment, if the endocrine therapy first chosen is inefficient while patients with "receptor-poor" or testosterone insensitive tumors, alternative forms of therapy should be offered, e.g. irradiation or cytotoxic drugs [155,157,158].

Most investigators in this field underline the potential value of these measurements as possible tumor marker for evaluating tumor testosterone dependence and, in turn, planning patients management and indicate a potential clinical usefulness for testosterone receptor analysis in the cure of patients with prostate cancer [155,159].

From the values listed in Table (3-5), there were a significant increase ($P < 0.1$) in the maximum number of binding sites (B_{max}) for malignant nuclear receptors compared with that of benign type. These results are inconsistent with those reported previously, Schröder and de Voogt (1980) with other investigators reported that androgen receptor levels were ranged from 0 to 110 fmole/mg DNA in benign tumors and ranged from 0 to 190 fmole/mg DNA in malignant tumors[155].

Ekman et al (1979) reported that the maximum binding sites (B_{max}) of androgen receptor in 25 cases of primary prostatic carcinoma varied between 7.7 and 73.8 fmole/mg protein and the K_a between 1.1 and 6.7×10^{10} M^{-1} [158].

Table (3-5): Concentrations and affinity constants of nuclear testosterone receptors in benign and malignant prostatic tumors. All details are described in section (2.5.2).

Group	Age (year)	Temp. (°C)	Binding capacity		K_a (× 10^{10} M^{-1})
			Fmole / mg protein	Fmole / mg DNA	
Benign prostatic hyperplasia	65.96±1.15	4	11.40	6.33	8.7
		10	11.55	6.38	9.35
		25	11.67	6.44	11.32
		37	11.78	6.50	12.80
		45	7.50	4.17	12.17
Prostatic adenocarcinoma	73.66±0.62	4	12.0	4	7.64
		10	12.3	4.11	8.79
		25	13.2	4.40	11.10
		37	13.4	4.47	13.12
		45	4.66	1.56	41.94

3.3.1.2. Determination of kinetic parameters of ^{125}I-testosterone binding to its nuclear receptors in human benign and malignant prostatic tumors

The time course of ^{125}I-testosterone binding to its benign and malignant receptors in prostatic tumors was carried out to describe the kinetic parameters of the binding.

The simplest proposed model representing the interaction of ^{125}I-testosterone with its receptors could be expressed by the following equation:

$$^{125}\text{I-testosterone} + R \underset{k_{-1}}{\overset{k_{+1}}{\rightleftharpoons}} {}^{125}\text{I-testosterone-R}$$

Where k_{+1} is the rate of the association of ^{125}I-testosterone with its receptors and k_{-1} represents the rate of the reverse reaction i.e., the dissociation of the complex formed under the same conditions:

At equilibrium;

$$k_a = \frac{[^{125}\text{I} - \text{testosterone} - \text{R}]}{[^{125}\text{I} - \text{testosterone}][\text{R}]} \tag{1}$$

$$k_d = \frac{[^{125}\text{I} - \text{testosterone}][\text{R}]}{[^{125}\text{I} - \text{testosterone} - \text{R}]} \tag{2}$$

Thus; $k_a = \dfrac{1}{k_d} = \dfrac{k_{+1}}{k_{-1}}$ $\tag{3}$

Where K_a is the equilibrium constant of the association (affinity constant) and k_d is the equilibrium constant of the dissociation of ^{125}I-testosterone-R complex.

The values of k_a and maximal binding capacity (B_{max}) were calculated from Scatchard plot at five different temperatures in Figure (3-17) and Table (3-5).

Results in Table (3-6) show that k_a value at 37°C for benign tumors is about 1.47 times that of k_a value at 4°C and the k_a value of malignant tumors at 45°C is about 5.48 times that of at 4°C.

The values of k_d calculated by using equation (3) show that the lowest k_d value of ^{125}I-testosterone-receptor complex occurs at 37°C for benign receptors and at 45°C for malignant receptors. Also, it was found that in temperatures from 4 to 25°C, the affinity of testosterone to its benign receptor was greater than that of malignant receptors while in temperatures from 37 to 45°C, the affinity of testosterone to its malignant receptors was greater than that of benign receptors. These results are in accordance with that obtained by previous study on rat prostate carcinoma (Dunning R-3327) which reported that binding of testosterone was of high affinity with its cytosolic receptor ($k_a = 2 \times 10^9$ M^{-1}) [144] and significantly different from those obtained previously [38,115,158,160] and these differences may be attributed to the differences in experimental methodology used, the differences in tissue sources and to differences in the structure of these receptors.

Table (3-6): The kinetic parameters of ^{125}I-testosterone binding to its receptors in benign and malignant prostatic tumors. All details are described in sections (2.5.1) and (2.5.2).

Temp. (°C)	Benign receptors			Malignant receptors		
	Binding capacity (fmole /mg protein)	$k_a = \dfrac{k_{+1}}{k_{-1}}$ $\times 10^{10}$(M^{-1})	$k_d = \dfrac{k_{-1}}{k_{+1}}$ $\times 10^{-12}$(M)	Binding capacity (fmole /mg protein)	$k_a = \dfrac{k_{+1}}{k_{-1}}$ $\times 10^{10}$(M^{-1})	$k_d = \dfrac{k_{-1}}{k_{+1}}$ $\times 10^{-12}$(M)
4	11.40	8.70	11.494	12.0	7.64	13.089
10	11.55	9.35	10.695	12.3	8.79	11.376
25	11.67	11.32	8.834	13.2	11.10	9.009
37	11.78	12.80	7.812	13.4	13.12	7.622
45	7.50	12.17	8.217	4.66	41.94	2.384

The kinetic association rate constant, k_{+1}, can be determined from the time course of association of ^{125}I-testosterone with its receptors and verified the order of the reaction at five different temperatures by using the following equations:

The integrated second order kinetics,

$$\ln \frac{(HR)_e((H)_T - (HR)_t (HR)_e/(R)_T)}{(H)_T[(HR)_e - (HR)_t]} = k_{+1}t\left[\frac{(H)_T(R)_T}{(HR)_e} - (HR)_e\right] \qquad (4)$$

Where $(H)_T$ is the total concentration of ^{125}I-testosterone, $(R)_T$ is the total concentration of binding sites, $(HR)_e$ is the concentration of testosterone–receptor complex at equilibrium, $(HR)_t$ is the concentration of testosterone–receptor complex at time (t) [161].

Or by using another second order kinetic equation form:

$$\frac{1}{S_o - Q_o}\ln\left(\frac{S_o - B_{(t)}}{Q_o - B_{(t)}}\right) = k_{+1}t + \frac{1}{S_o - Q_o}\ln\frac{S_o}{Q_o} \qquad (5)$$

Where S_o is the total concentration of ^{125}I-testosterone, Q_o is the total concentration of receptor binding sites, B(t) is the concentration of specifically bound testosterone at time (t) and k_{+1} is the association rate constant [162].

Equation (4) could be simplified to equation (6) when the most testosterone remained free and only a small fraction of $(H)_T$ is bound even at equilibrium (pseudo-first order conditions) [161].

$$\ln \frac{(HR)_e}{(HR)_e - (HR)_t} = k_{+1}t\left[\frac{(H)_T (R)_T}{(HR)_e}\right] \tag{6}$$

The time course data obtained from Figure (3-16 A&B) could be used to confirm that the binding reaction of testosterone with its benign prostatic receptors following a second order kinetic reactions at temperatures (4,10,25,37 and 45°C).

For this purpose, $\dfrac{1}{S_o - Q_o}\ln\left(\dfrac{S_o - B_{(t)}}{Q_o - B_{(t)}}\right)$ was plotted against time (t) as shown in Figure (3-18), k_{+1} was determined at each temperature from the slope of the plot, while malignant prostatic tumor receptors interactions with testosterone obey pseudo-first order kinetic at 4,10,25,37, and 45°C, thus equation (6) was used.

Figure (3-19) shows that the plotting of $\ln \dfrac{(HR)_e}{(HR)_e - (HR)_t}$ against time (t) gives a straight line with a slope equal to the observed value of first-order rate constant $(k_{obs.})$ in min^{-1}, and the association rate constant k_{+1} was calculated from the following formula:

$$k_{obs.} = k_{+1}\frac{(H)_T (R)_T}{(HR)_e} \tag{7}$$

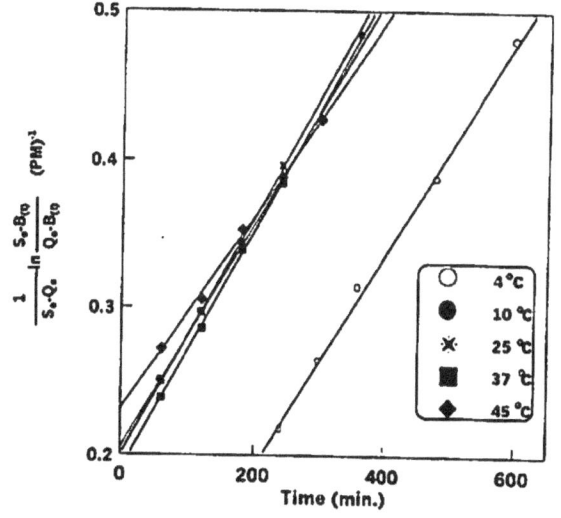

Figure (3-18): Second order kinetics of ^{125}I-testosterone binding with its benign prostatic receptors at different temperatures. All details are described in section (2.5.1).

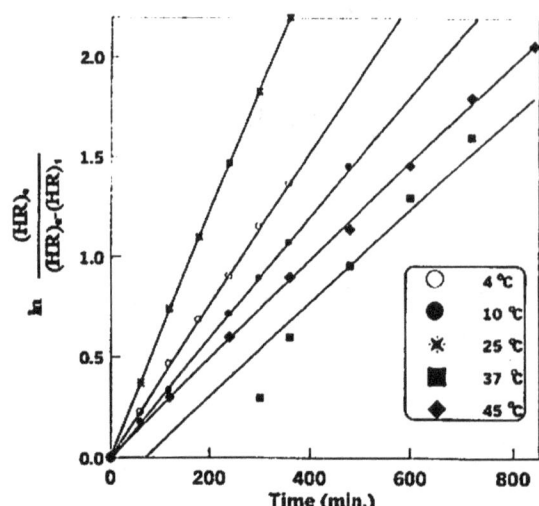

Figure (3–19): Pseudo-first order kinetics of ^{125}I-testosterone binding with its malignant prostatic receptors at different temperatures. All details are described in section (2.5.1).

The half-life time of association $(t_{1/2})_{ass.}$, which represents the time needed for the formation of half amount of the complex at equilibrium, was determined from the concentration of the complex at equilibrium and the time course curve. While the half-life time of dissociation $(t_{1/2})_{diss.}$ was determined from:

$$\left(t_{1/2}\right)_{diss} = \frac{\ln 2}{k-1} = \frac{0.693}{k-1} \tag{8}$$

For first order reaction kinetics, and from:

$$\left(t_{1/2}\right)_{diss} = \frac{1}{k-1(Q_o)} \tag{9}$$

For second order reaction kinetics.

The results revealed that the association rate constant k_{+1} at 37°C was higher than that of at 4°C by approximately 1.2 fold for benign tumors while, the k_{+1} value at 45°C was higher than that of 4°C by approximately 4.4 fold for malignant tumors and also it was found that k_{+1} values at 4,10,25 and 37°C for benign tumors were significantly higher than that of malignant tumors at each temperature. This may be attributed to the high extent of association between ^{125}I-testosterone with its benign receptors compared with malignant receptors at the same temperatures. The k_{-1} values were determined from the equation (3).

Table (3-7) shows that k_{-1} decreased with the elevation of temperature. Thus when the reaction temperature was increased from 4°C to 37°C, the value of the dissociation constant decreased approximately 1.3 fold for benign and malignant tumors receptors. Previous study on rat prostate carcinoma (Dunning R-3327) reported that rate of testosterone dissociation from its receptors were slow ($t_{1/2}$= 60 hrs) [163]. This numerical difference may be attributed to the different types of receptor sources used.

Table (3-7): The effect of temperature on the kinetic parameters of testosterone binding to its receptors in benign and malignant prostatic tumors. All details are described in section (2.5.1).

Temp. (°C)	Benign receptors					Malignant receptors				
	k_{+1} (M.min)$^{-1}$ ×10^{5}	k_{-1} (min^{-1}) ×10^{-4}	$(t_{1/2})_{ass}$ (hr)	$(t_{1/2})_{diss}$ (PM^{-1} hr)	k_{a} (M^{-1}) ×10^{10}	k_{+1} (M.min)$^{-1}$ ×10^{5}	k_{-1} (min^{-1}) ×10^{-4}	$(t_{1/2})_{ass}$ (hr)	$(t_{1/2})_{diss}$ (hr)	k_{a} (M^{-1}) ×10^{10}
4	7.332	84.276	3.1	0.86	8.7	1.366	17.879	2.700	6.46	7.64
10	7.511	80.331	1.8	0.90	9.35	1.461	16.621	2.66	6.95	8.79
25	7.896	69.752	1.75	1.03	11.32	1.664	14.990	2.20	7.70	11.10
37	8.224	64.25	1.66	1.10	12.8	1.784	13.597	2.16	8.49	13.12
45	6.477	53.221	3.70	2.08	12.17	6.074	14.483	2.14	16.44	41.935

3.3.1.3. Estimation of Hill coefficients (n) of nuclear testosterone receptors in human benign and malignant prostatic tumors

On application of the Hill equation, it would be possible to evaluate the cooperativity of the binding sites of testosterone receptors through the determination of Hill coefficient (n). Figure (3–20 A&B) represents the Hill plots of ^{125}I-testosterone binding to its nuclear prostatic receptors in benign and malignant prostatic tumors at different temperatures.

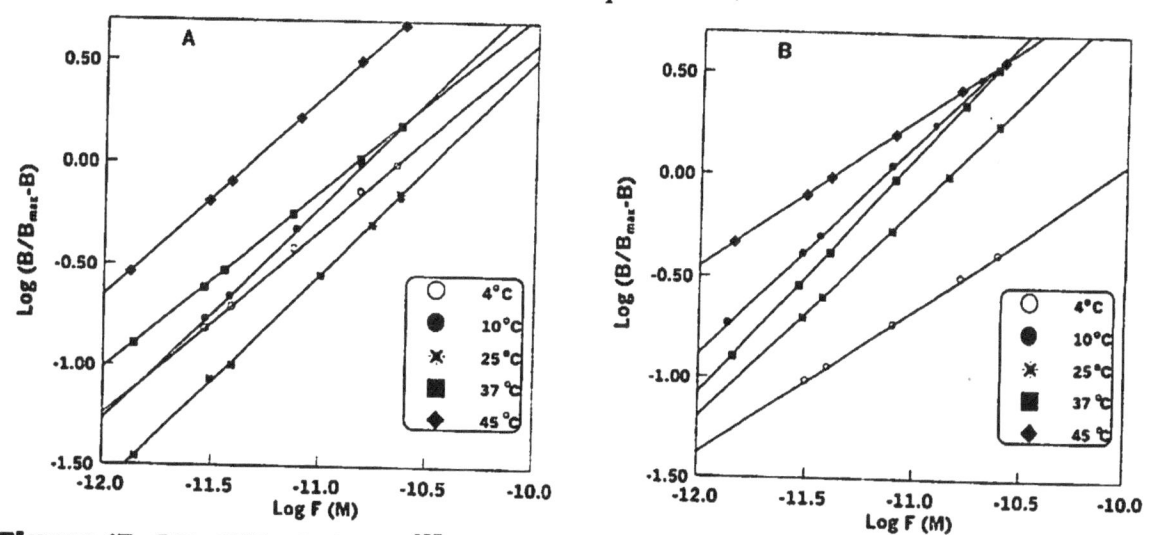

Figure (3–20): Hill plots of ^{125}I-testosterone binding to its nuclear receptors from, A) benign prostatic tumors, B) malignant prostatic tumors, at five different temperatures. All details are described in section (2.5.3).

The results listed in Table (3-8) revealed that the Hill coefficients were equal to 1 and no significant differences were found between the results obtained for benign and those obtained for malignant receptors, suggesting that there were no cooperativity between testosterone binding sites on testosterone receptor molecule during the binding reaction with testosterone.

Table (3-8): Effect of temperature on the binding sites cooperativity of testosterone receptors in benign and malignant prostatic tumors. All details are described in sections (2.5.3).

Temp. (°C)	Hill coefficients Benign receptors	Hill coefficients Malignant receptors
4	0.937	0.714
10	1.055	1.021
25	1.077	1.077
37	0.875	1.180
45	0.972	0.732

3.3.2. The thermodynamics of the binding of ^{125}I-testosterone to its receptors in benign and malignant prostatic tumors

3.3.2.1. Thermodynamic parameters of standard state

Figure (3–21) represents the dependence of the equilibrium binding constant (i.e., affinity constant) for the binding of ^{125}I-testosterone to its receptors in prostatic tumor homogenate on the temperature (Van't Hoff plot).

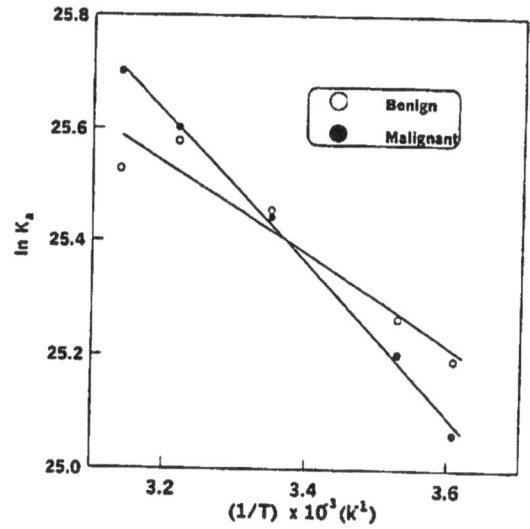

Figure (3-21): Van't Hoff plot for the ^{125}I-testosterone binding to its prostatic receptors. All details are described in section (2.5.4).

The results indicated that ΔH^o in general had small values and nearly close to zero, their positive sign ascertain that the reaction were nearly endothermic. The ΔH^o value in the case of malignant receptors was higher than that in the case of benign receptors, so more energy is needed in case of malignant receptors for the reaction (binding) to occur.

The negative values of ΔG^o reflect the stability of the complex hence, the high affinity of the reactants. The high negative values of ΔG^o for the binding reactions are controlled by high positive ΔS^o values as shwon in Table (3-9). So, our system is characterized by the sole contribution of ΔS^o to the stability of the complexes formed, while ΔH^o has little or no effect.

A high value of positive ΔS^o suggests that the reaction spontaneity was entropically driven. Entropy was the driven force for the occurrence of the binding reaction. Table (3-9) showed that ΔH^o and ΔS^o values for the binding of ^{125}I-testosterone to its malignant prostatic receptors were higher than those for benign receptors, this means that binding of ^{125}I-testosterone with its malignant receptors needs more energy, and the complex formed (product) possessed a less ordered structure than the reactant species, i.e. ^{125}I-testosterone and testosterone receptors.

The small positive ΔH^o may indicate a favorable interaction between groups within both testosterone and its receptors. These include the non-covalent interactions which are fundamentally electrostatic in nature such as charge–charge interactions which occurs in both testosterone and its receptors in prostatic tumor homogenate, other types of interactions include charge-dipole, dipole-dipole, charge–induced dipole, dipole–induced dipole and hydrogen bond. The sum of these types of interactions can yield some stabilization to the folded structure of the complex. So, the negative value of ΔG^0 showed that the overall reaction was energetically favorable in the direction of complex formation.

The results listed in Table (3-9) indicate that the reaction spontaneity for malignant receptors was smaller than that for benign receptors at optimum temperature [164-166]. Also, it was concluded that short range interactions including Van der Waals' interactions, protonations and hydrogen bond formation were more important factors in stabilizing the malignant receptor complex than that of benign receptors.

Table (3-9): Thermodynamic parameters at standard state of testosterone binding to its receptors in benign and malignant prostatic tumors. All details are described in section (2.5.4).

Temp. (°C)	Benign receptors			Malignant receptors		
	ΔH^0 (kJ/mole)	ΔG^0 (kJ/mole)	ΔS^0 (J/mole.K)	ΔH^0 (kJ/mole)	ΔG^0 (kJ/mole)	ΔS^0 (J/mole.K)
4	+8.31441	-58.013	+239.449	+11.877	-57.713	+251.227
10	+8.31441	-59.439	+239.417	+11.877	-59.293	+251.484
25	+8.31441	-63.063	+239.521	+11.877	-63.014	+251.312
37	+8.31441	-65.919	+239.462	+11.877	-65.983	+251.161
45	+8.31441	-67.487	+238.369	+11.877	-70.758	+259.858

3.3.2.2. Thermodynamic parameters of Transition State

According to the transition state theory, the interaction of testosterone with its receptor leads to the formation of an activated complex (transition state), then the formation of the final product:

Testosterone + R ⟶ [Testosterone-R] * ⟶ Testosterone-R

An activated complex   Final product
(Transition state)

The transition state thermodynamic parameters ΔH^*, ΔG^*, ΔS^*, E_a and Q_{10} could be determined from Arrhenius equation.

Figure (3–22) shows the dependence of the association rate for the binding of ^{125}I-testosterone to its receptors in prostatic tumor homogenate on temperature (Arrhenius plot).

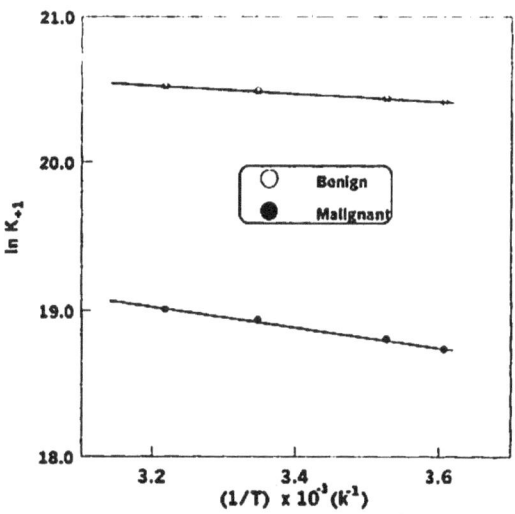

Figure (3–22): Arrhenius plot for the ^{125}I-testosterone binding to its prostatic receptors. All details are described in section (2.5.4).

The high positive value of ΔG^* indicated that the formation of an activated [testosterone-R] complex was a non spontaneous process and required a lot of energy (equal to E_a) to overcome the transition state energy barrier and giving the final product, whereas the high negative ΔS^* revealed that the activated complex had a more ordered structure than the reactant species ($\Delta S^* < 0$). The positive values of ΔG^* is mainly attributed to the decrease in entropy of the transition state ($\Delta S^* < 0$). In addition, the positive value of ΔH^* shows that the heat content of the activated complex is more than that of isolated species [167]. The results in Table (3-10) show that the values of E_a and ΔH^* for the binding reactions of testosterone with its malignant prostatic receptors were more than that in the case of benign receptors and the E_a value for malignant receptors was greater than that of benign receptors by a factor of 2.40. Therefore, the binding reaction of testosterone with benign receptors was easy to occur when compared with the same reaction with malignant receptors. The negative values of ΔS^* for malignant receptors were slightly greater than that of benign receptors, so it was concluded that hydrophobic interactions may play an important role in stabilizing the malignant receptor activated complex formed.

The effect of temperature on the rate of binding reaction is frequently expressed in terms of a temperature coefficient, Q_{10}, which is the factor by which the rate increases by raising the temperature 10°C. Table (3-11) shows the Q_{10} values of the interaction between testosterone and its receptors at different temperature ranges.

The Q_{10} values of benign receptors were smaller than that of malignant receptors at the same temperature ranges, this may reflect that the binding of testosterone with benign receptors has been stimulated to proceed more than that with malignant receptors. Most references pointed to that Q_{10} values usually has a value in the region of 1-2 [110,111].

Table (3-10): Thermodynamic parameters at transition state of testosterone binding to its receptors in benign and malignant prostatic tumors. All details are described in section (2.5.4).

Temp. (°C)	Benign receptors				Malignant receptors			
	E_a (kJ/mole)	ΔH^* (kJ/mole)	ΔG^* (kJ/mole)	ΔS^* (J/mole.K)	E_a (kJ/mole)	ΔH^* (kJ/mole)	ΔG^* (kJ/mole)	ΔS^* (J/mole.K)
4	2.690	0.387	20.662	-73.195	6.466	4.163	24.532	-73.534
10	2.690	0.337	21.103	-73.378	6.466	4.113	24.956	-73.650
25	2.690	0.213	22.226	-73.869	6.466	3.989	26.084	-74.144
37	2.690	0.113	23.118	-74.210	6.466	3.889	27.057	-74.735
45	2.690	0.047	24.414	-76.626	6.466	3.823	24.584	-65.286

Table (3-11): Temperature coefficients (Q_{10}) for the binding of ^{125}I-testosterone with its benign and malignant prostatic tumors receptors. All details are described in section (2.5.4).

Temp. range (°C)	Q_{10} value Benign receptors	Q_{10} value Malignant receptors
0–10	1.042	1.106
10–20	1.039	1.098
20–30	1.037	1.091
30–40	1.034	1.085
40–50	1.032	1.080

Determination of the thermodynamic parameters of the binding reaction using equilibrium data gives an overall idea about the nature of forces controlling complex formation. Comparison of the values of transition state with those of standard state in Tables (3-9) and (3-10) led us to choose a thermodynamic model shown in Figure (3–23). Our model proposes that the formation of the ^{125}I-testosterone-receptor complex undergoes three thermodynamic states. Thermodynamic state A represents the initial energy level of the isolated ^{125}I-testosterone and its receptor (R). In thermodynamic state B, the two components have come together and mutually penetrated their hydration sphere to form a partially immobilized hydrophobically associated species. Thermodynamic state C represents the fully interacting complex (^{125}I-testosterone-R). In step 1 of the reaction, the binding of ^{125}I-testosterone to its receptor was associated with positive ΔG^* value. This indicates that the initial step of the reaction requires input of energy for the system. The negative entropy change ΔS^* for this step of the reaction reflects the change of the ^{125}I-testosterone-R transition complex to a more ordered structure. The positive ΔH^* value shows that the heat content of the activated complex is more than that of the isolated species. Partial immobilization of the hydrophobically associated complex formed, in step1, occurs when isolated hydrated species ^{125}I-testosterone and receptor (R) interact partially so that there is a mutual penetration of their hydration layers to form the activated complex. This hydrophobic association is a result of the tendency of water to form a more ordered structure in the vicinity of non-polar hydrocarbon groups (eg., the side chains of the amino acids phenylalanine, leucine and tryptophan) this means that hydrophobic amino acid side chains which were previously accessible to solvent in the isolated species become buried upon complex formation. In step 2, the activated complex participates in further interactions, giving the fully interacting complex (^{125}I-testosterone-R). It is proposed that the formation of a testosterone-receptor complex occurs in two steps, the first step stabilized the complex by hydrophobic interactions and the second step stabilized it by short range interactions such as electrostatic interactions, hydrogen bonding and Van der Waals' interactions [168].

Hydrophobic interactions contribute to the stability of the complex via large decrease in the excited entropy change ($\Delta S^* < 0$), while electrostatic interactions, hydrogen bonding and Van der Waals' interactions stabilize the complex via high increase in the standard entropy change ($\Delta S° > 0$) [168,169].

The thermodynamic data from this study indicate that the binding of ^{125}I-testosterone to its receptors are entropically driven and come in agreement with the concept that hydrophobic and short-range interactions have an important role in the binding of testosterone to its malignant prostatic receptors rather than that with benign receptors.

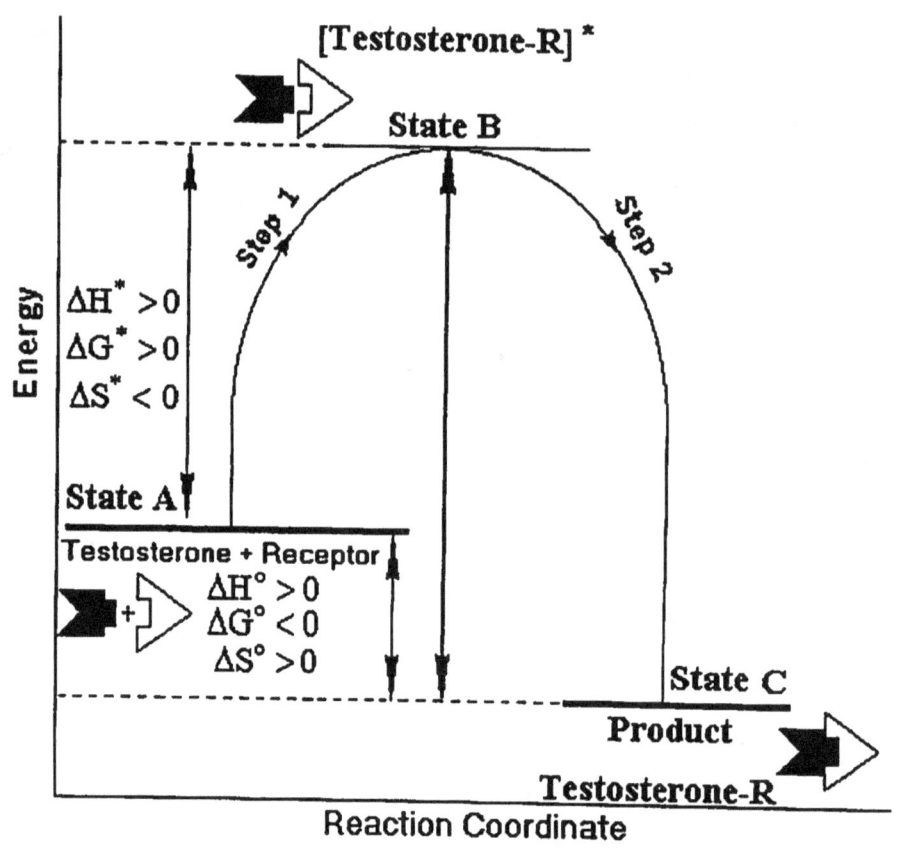

Figure (3–23): General energy diagram and thermodynamic model applied to the interaction of ^{125}I-testosterone with its nuclear receptors in prostatic tumors.

3.4. Purification and isolation of nuclear testosterone receptors using gel filtration technique

Purification and isolation of nuclear testosterone receptors were performed by gel exclusion chromatography technique. Benign and malignant homogenates were applied to sephadex G-200 (0.7×28 cm) column. The void volume of this column was 6 ml as predicted from the elution profile of the blue dextran as shown in Figure (3–24 A). The resultant fractions of each homogenate type were collected, detected for the binding with ^{125}I-testosterone as described in sections (2.6.4) and (2.6.5), pooled, concentrated and then subjected to protein determination as mentioned in section (2.3.1). This experiment revealed as shown in Figure (3–24 B&C) the presence of two different eluted components (I & II), these two components eluted with different elution volume corresponding to their different molecular weights. From benign tumors homogenate, the first one (BI) eluted with the void volume (V_o) while the second one (BII) eluted with about 2.5 V_o. From malignant tumors homogenate, (MI) eluted with one fraction after the void volume (V_o) while the second one (MII) eluted with 2.5 V_o.

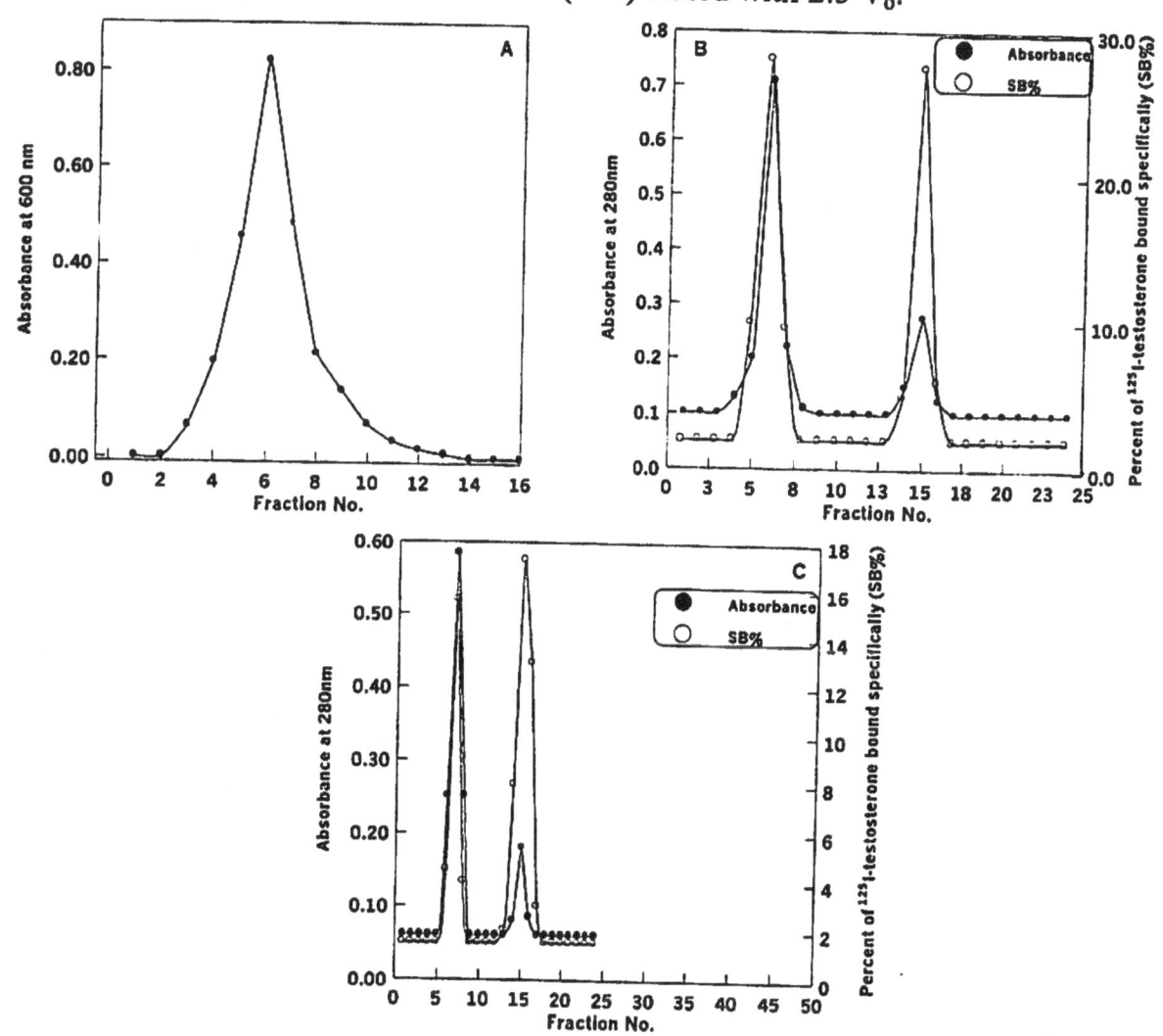

Figure (3–24): Elution profiles of: A) Blue dextran 2000, B) testosterone receptors from BPH homogenate, C) testosterone receptors from PCA homogenate. All details are described in section (2.6).

From these results, it was concluded that these components are capable of binding to the testosterone with different affinities and in general receptors type II have higher affinities for the binding than those of receptors type (I). The first eluted component (I) with a higher molecular weight is an aggregated complex of testosterone receptor and nuclear matrix. The nuclear matrix is a chromatin-depleted and salt-washable, proteinaceous (non-histonic), intra-nuclear structure or may be defined as nuclear scaffolding proteins which provide functional organization for DNA. Many biological functions reported to be associated with the nuclear matrix include steroid hormone binding, DNA-replication sites, RNA synthesis and processing.

In the last two decades, great interest has developed in the molecular characterization of the matrix bound androgen receptors in the normal and diseased prostate glands of different species and different ligand used[65,115,170,171].

An indication of such complex formation is available from previous studies by Mainwaring, Irving and others [65,138,172,173].

The second component (II) represents the purified testosterone receptors with a lower molecular weight than the first one (about 110 kDa) [174,175]. Table (3-12) illustrates the purification parameters for the different purified receptor forms isolated by gel exclusion chromatography technique. The elution profiles result from the experiment as shown in Figure (3-24 B&C) were nearly similar to that obtained previously by many investigators worked mainly on rat prostate[142,153,131,176-186].

Table (3-12): Purification data of testosterone receptors isolated by gel filtration technique. All details are described in section (2.6).

Receptor type	Total proteins (μgm)	Specifically bound ^{125}I-testosterone (fM)	Specific binding Fmole ^{125}I-testosterone /mg protein	Purification factor (fold)
Crude benign prostatic tumors homogenate	250	3.480	13.920	1.000
BI purified fraction	200	32.261	161.308	11.588
BII purified fraction	100	27.258	272.586	19.582
Crude malignant prostatic tumors homogenate	100	1.110	11.100	1.000
MI purified fraction	85	22.908	269.515	24.280
MII purified fraction	70	22.620	323.143	29.111

3.5. The Choice of most appropriate conditions of ^{125}I-testosterone binding to its purified nuclear receptors

3.5.1. The effect of different concentrations of testosterone receptors on the binding with ^{125}I-testosterone

Figure (3–25) shows the effect of increasing amounts of purified receptors on the binding with ^{125}I-testosterone. The results revealed that 250µgm protein was the most appropriate concentration of the binding of BI and MI purified fractions while 200 µgm of protein for BII purified fraction and 150 µgm protein was the most appropriate concentration of the binding of MII purified fraction. From these results, it could be concluded that the binding of ^{125}I-testosterone with its purified receptors BII and MII needed lower amounts of these receptors to get the equilibrium compared with the amounts required for BI and MI purified receptors. This may be due to cell hyperproliferation or increase in these receptors affinities for testosterone.

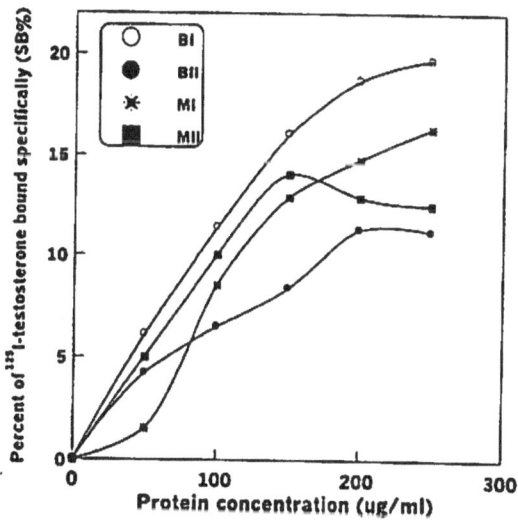

Figure (3–25): The effect of protein concentration on ^{125}I-testosterone binding to its purified nuclear receptors. All details are described in section (2.7.1).

3.5.2. The choice of most appropriate concentration of ^{125}I-testosterone for the binding with its purified nuclear receptors

Figure (3–26) shows that purified nuclear receptors were saturated with testosterone concentrations equal to 72.498 PM for BI purified fraction, 57.997 PM for BII, MI purified fractions and 43.5 PM for MII purified fraction. From these results, it was found that BII and MII purified fractions were saturated with smaller concentrations of ^{125}I-testosterone than these required for BI and MI. Thus it was concluded that BII and MII purified receptors have higher affinities (but not concentrations) toward testosterone than BI and MI purified fractions.

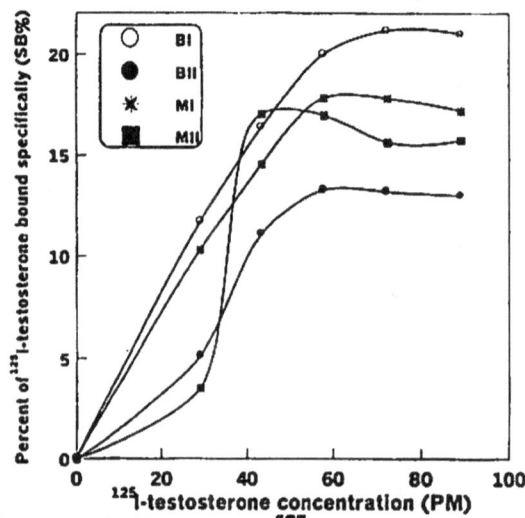

Figure (3–26): The effect of different ^{125}I-testosterone concentrations on the binding to its purified nuclear receptors. All details are described in section (2.7.2).

3.5.3. The effect of different pH on the binding of ^{125}I-testosterone with its purified nuclear receptors

Figure (3–27) shows the effect of increasing pH on the binding of ^{125}I-testosterone to its purified receptors. The results revealed that the optimum pH for BI and MII purified fractions for the binding with testosterone was 7.8 while 7 was the optimum pH for the binding of testosterone with MI purified receptor and 8.6 for BII purified receptor binding with testosterone.

These differences in the optimum pHs may suggest the differences in the binding sites of these purified receptors [110]. Also it was found that BII purified receptor binding site contains basic amino acid residues more than that of MII purified receptor.

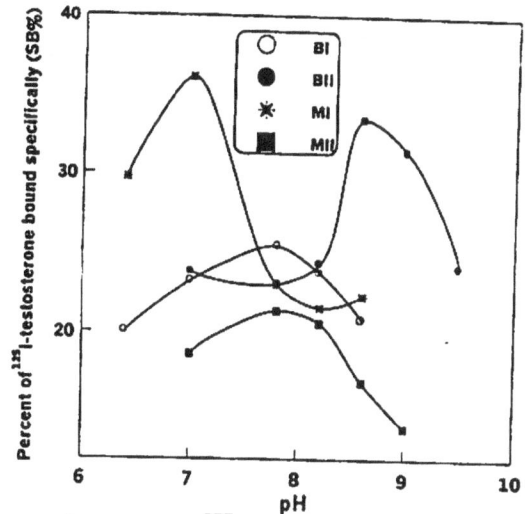

Figure (3–27): pH dependency of ^{125}I-testosterone binding with its purified nuclear receptors. All details are described in section (2.7.3).

3.5.4. The effect of incubation time on the binding of ^{125}I-testosterone with its purified nuclear receptors

Figure (3–28) shows that at 37°C the apparent equilibria of the ^{125}I-testosterone binding were reached in 2 hrs for BI purified receptor, 10 hrs for MI purified receptor, 6 hrs for BII and MII purified receptors.

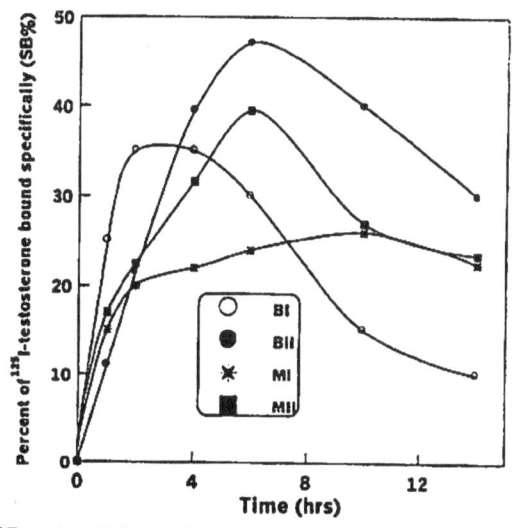

Figure (3–28): The effect of incubation time on the binding of ^{125}I-testosterone with its purified nuclear receptors. All details are described in section (2.7.4).

3.5.5. Temperature dependency of ^{125}I-testosterone binding to its purified nuclear receptors

The temperature dependency of the testosterone binding to its purified nuclear receptors was investigated. Figure (3–29) shows that the optimum temperature of the binding of ^{125}I-testosterone was 10°C with BI purified receptor, 25°C with BII purified receptor, 4°C for MI purified receptor and 45°C with MII purified receptor.

In general the loss of specific binding activity above the optimum temperature of BI, BII and MI purified receptors may be due to degradation of these receptor molecules or to the irreversible dissociation of the testosterone receptor complexes.

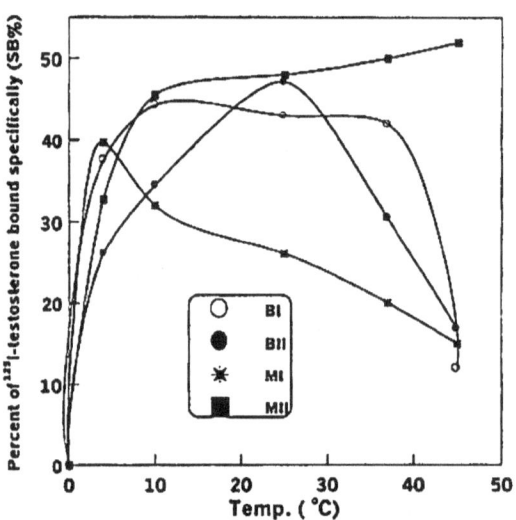

Figure (3–29): Effect of temperature on the binding of ^{125}I-testosterone with its purified nuclear receptors. All details are described in section (2.7.5).

3.6. The effect of anticancer drugs on the binding of ^{125}I-testosterone with its purified malignant nuclear receptors

Many investigators underlined that the most effective chemotherapies in treating hormone–resistant prostate cancer patients are cisplatin, vincristine sulfate, 5-fluorouracil and cyclophosphamide [5,15].

The experiment was carried out to explore the effect of these drugs on the binding of testosterone hormone with its receptors in human malignant prostatic tumors. These drugs were capable of inhibiting the binding of testosterone with its malignant receptors with different extent depending on the receptor and drug type. Figure (3-30) shows the inhibition percents of these drugs for the purified malignant nuclear receptors, from these results it was found that cisplatin and 5-fluorouracil have the greatest inhibiting effect than the other drugs.

Liao S. (1994) reported that some small molecules could bind to mutated androgen receptors and transactivate target genes by competing with testosterone for the binding [75]. The loss of androgen specificity of the nuclear receptors from prostatic cancer specimens was also reported by other investigators [37,33,74,96].

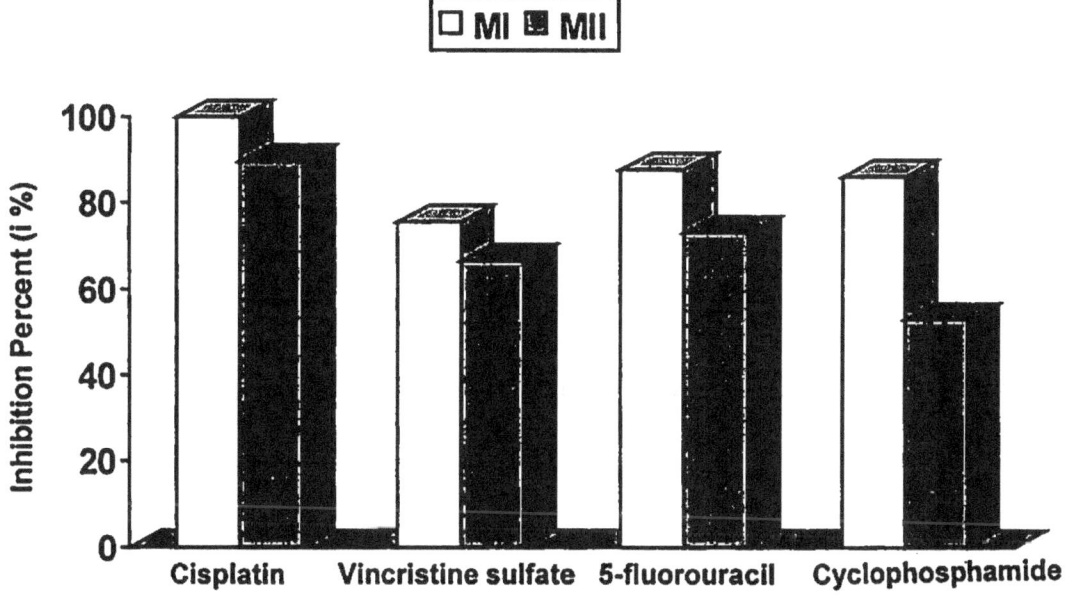

Figure (3–30): Inhibitory effects of different cytotoxic chemotherapy on the binding of ^{125}I-testosterone with its purified malignant nuclear receptors. All details are described in section (2.7.6).

3.7. The kinetics and thermodynamics of the interaction of testosterone with its purified nuclear receptors

3.7.1. Kinetics of the ^{125}I-testosterone binding to its purified receptors in benign and malignant prostatic tumors

Figure (3–31 A, B, C&D) shows the time course of the association of ^{125}I-testosterone with its purified nuclear receptor at different temperatures (4,10,25,37 and 45°C) in benign and malignant prostatic tumors. The concentration of ^{125}I-testosterone-receptor complex that formed after time (t) was calculated from the following equation:

$$[^{125}I - testosterone - receptor] in (PM) = \frac{\begin{array}{c} count\,(cpm)\,of\,^{125}I - testosterone \\ specifically\,bound\,after\,time\,(t) \end{array}}{\begin{array}{c} Total\,count\,(cpm)\,of\,^{125}I - testosterone \\ used\,in\,the\,incubation \end{array}} \times \left(\begin{array}{c} conc.\,of\,the \\ ^{125}I - testosterone \\ in\,the\,incubation \\ medium\,(PM) \end{array} \right)$$

The results of time course patterns at different temperatures revealed that the binding of testosterone to its purified nuclear receptors in prostatic tumors homogenate is a temperature and time dependent process with a maximum binding occurs at 10°C in 2 hrs for BI-purified receptor, 25°C in 6 hrs for BII-purified receptor, 4°C in 6 hrs for MI-purified receptor and at 45°C in 14 hrs for MII-purified receptor.

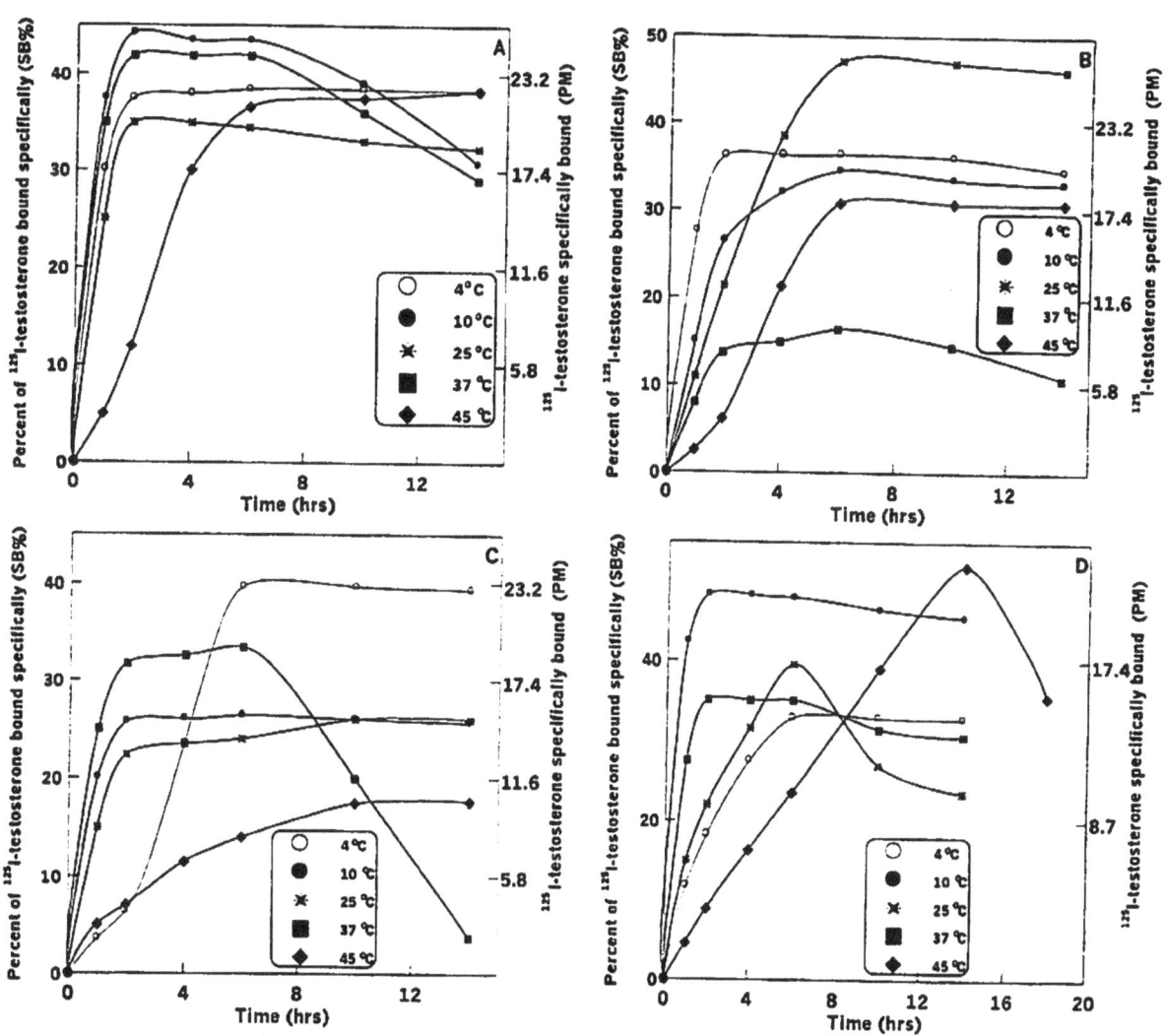

Figure (3-31): Time course of purified nuclear testosterone, A) BI-receptor, B) BII-receptor, C) MI-receptor, D) MII-receptor at different temperatures. All details are described in section (2.8.1).

3.7.1.1. Determination of the concentrations of purified nuclear testosterone receptors and the affinity constants of testosterone association with its purified nuclear receptors in human benign and malignant prostatic tumors

Scatchard plot analysis gave a straight line as shown in Figure (3-32 A, B, C&D) for each purified receptor at each temperature (4,10,25,37 and 45°C) indicating the presence of only a single class of receptor site, or more but with the same affinity and number of binding sites, these results were summarized in Table (3-13). Many reports indicate the possibility of using the nuclear testosterone receptor content as a possible marker of responsiveness to hormonal therapy in prostatic carcinoma [187,188].

Many investigators worked on rat prostate tumors reported that the concentration of matrix bound nuclear androgen receptors may represent the functional intranuclear androgen receptor in prostate cancer and characterization of these sites may also provide an understanding of the etiology of benign prostatic hyperplasia and cancer of the prostate. Possibly, the combined quantitation of testosterone receptor content and matrix-bound nuclear testosterone receptors is necessary for accurate prognosis and prediction of androgen-dependence of prostatic cancer specimens [65,115,170,171,187,189,190]. Gonor et al (1984), underlined that nuclear matrix bound androgen receptor could accurately identify those patients who should receive chemotherapy early in the progression of aggressive androgen-independent disease when the tumor burden is less, in the hope that this would increase both patient tolerance and tumor response to this treatment [171].

The results in Table (3-13) show that k_a value at 37°C for BII-purified receptor is about two times that of k_a value for BI-purified receptor while the k_a value at the same temperature for MII-purified receptor is about 8.5 times that of MI-purified receptor and about 20.2 times that of BI-purified receptor. In general, it was found that testosterone receptors interact with testosterone with higher affinity than the interaction of testosterone with nuclear matrix.

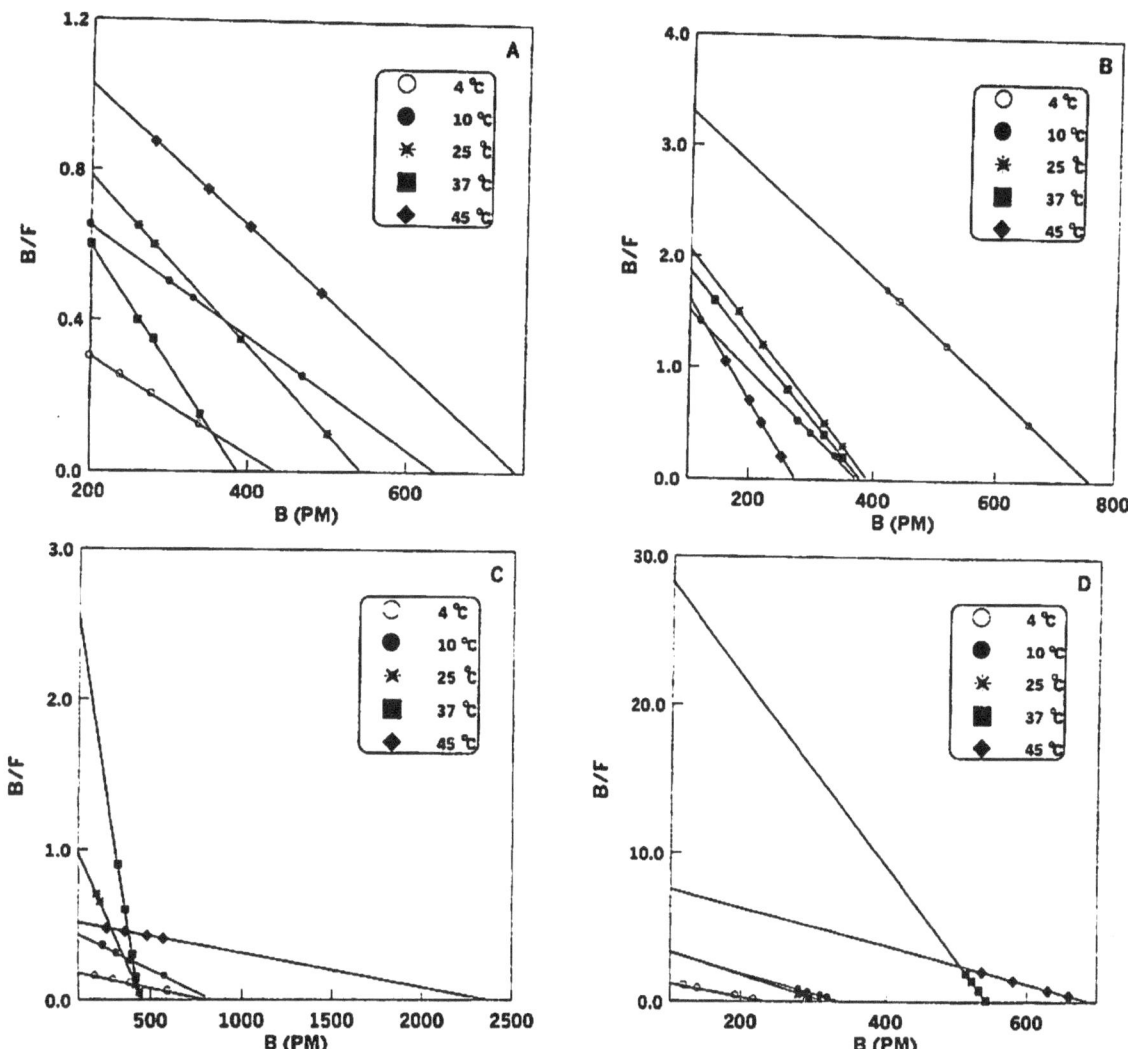

Figure (3–32): Scatchard plot of ^{125}**I-testosterone binding with its purified nuclear, A) BI-receptor, B) BII-receptor, C) MI-receptor, D) MII-receptor at different temperatures. All details are described in section (2.8.2).**

Table (3-13): Concentrations and affinity constants of purified nuclear testosterone receptors in benign and malignant prostatic tumors. All details are described in section (2.8.2).

Temp. (°C)	BI-purified receptor		BII-purified receptor		MI-purified receptor		MII-purified receptor	
	Binding capacity Pmole/mg protein	$k_a \times 10^{+9}$ (M^{-1})	Binding capacity Pmole/mg protein	$k_a \times 10^{+9}$ (M^{-1})	Binding capacity Pmole/mg protein	$k_a \times 10^{+9}$ (M^{-1})	Binding capacity Pmole/mg protein	$k_a \times 10^{+9}$ (M^{-1})
4	1.036	1.318	2.280	4.96	1.870	0.294	0.920	8.81
10	1.920	1.571	1.122	5.48	2.008	0.592	1.344	13.80
25	1.305	2.313	1.173	7.04	1.099	2.792	1.183	34.00
37	0.931	3.211	1.140	6.69	1.056	7.590	2.163	65.10
45	1.757	1.922	0.822	9.38	1.466	0.229	2.768	12.50

3.7.1.2. Determination of kinetic parameters of ^{125}I-testosterone binding to its purified nuclear receptors

The time course of ^{125}I-testosterone binding to its purified receptors in benign and malignant prostatic tumors was carried out to calculate the kinetic parameters of the binding. The time course data obtained from Figure (3–31 A, B, C&D) could be used to confirm that the reaction of testosterone with its benign and malignant purified receptors obeys pseudo-first order kinetics as shown in Figure (3–33 A, B, C&D). The results listed in Table (3-14) were nearly similar to that obtained previously by Lea and French who reported that binding of testosterone with its receptor in rat prostatic carcinoma (Dunning R-3327) was of high affinity $\left(k_a = 2 \times 10^9 M^{-1}\right)$ and rates of dissociation were slow ($t_{1/2} = 60$ hrs) [163]. It was found that MII-purified receptor has the same kinetic parameters in human and rat prostate cancer. As a result, this may reflect the high similarity of MII-purified receptor in human prostate gland with testosterone receptor in rat prostate cancer. Also the results of this work of B_{max}, k_a and $t_{1/2}$ values are in accordance with those reported previously [154, 38, 145, 191].

Finally, it was found that k_{+1} value increased with the elevation of temperature. Thus when the reaction temperature was increased from 4°C to 37°C, the value of the association rate constant increased approximately 2.8 fold for BI-purified receptor, 2 fold for BII and MII-purified receptors and 3.1 fold for MI-purified receptor.

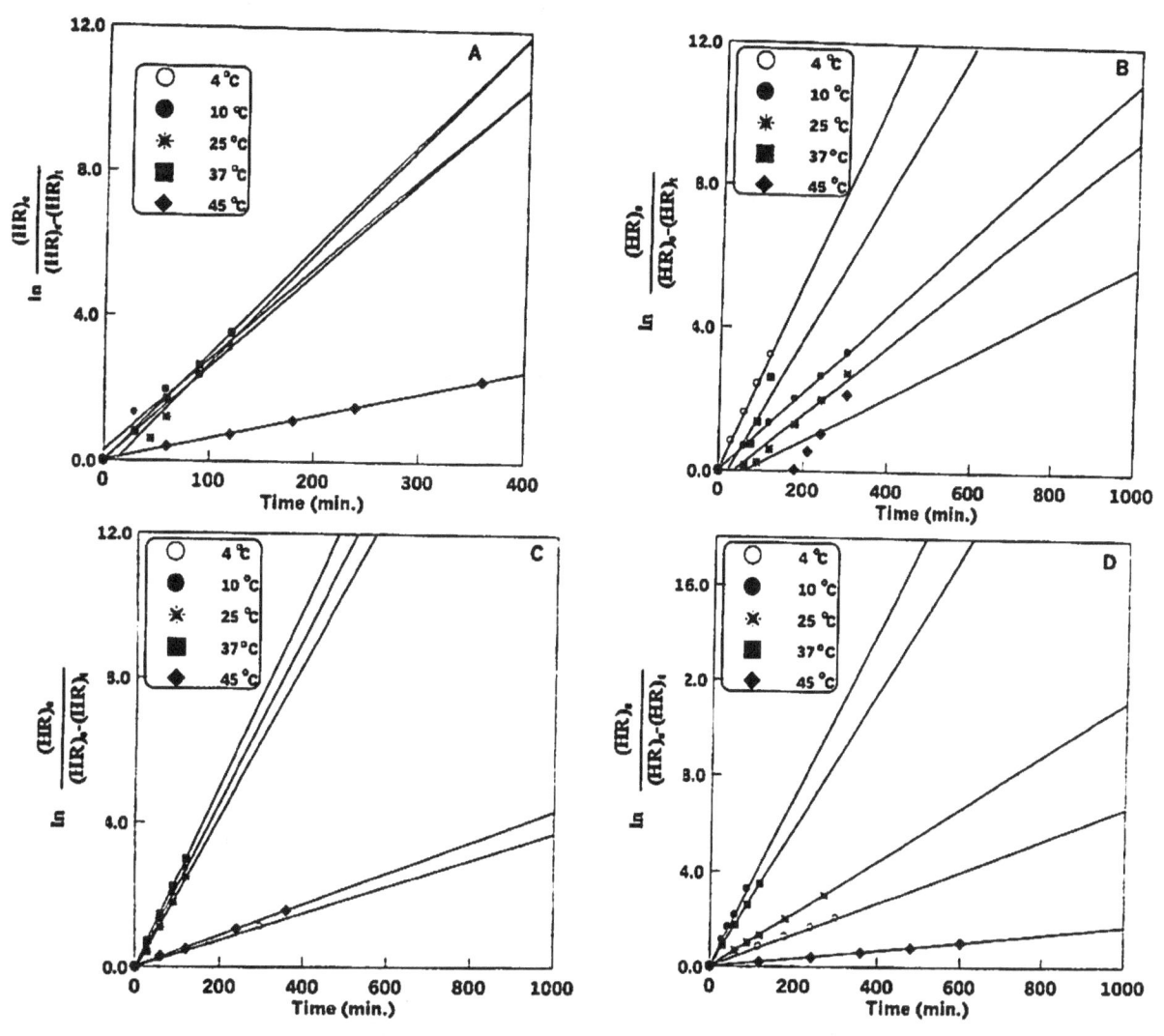

Figure (3-33): Pseudo-first order kinetics of ^{125}I-testosterone binding with its purified nuclear, A) BI-receptor, B) BII-receptor, C) MI-receptor, D) MII-receptor at different temperatures. All details are described in section (2.8.1).

Table (3-14): The effect of temperature on the kinetic parameters of testosterone binding to its purified nuclear receptors. All details are described in sections (2.8.1) and (2.8.2).

Purified receptor	Kinetic parameter	4°C	10°C	25°C	37°C	45°C
BI	$k_a \times 10^9 (M^{-1})$	1.318	1.571	2.313	3.211	1.922
	$k_d \times 10^{-9} (M)$	0.758	0.636	0.432	0.311	0.520
	$k_{+1} \times 10^7 (M^{-1}.min^{-1})$	1.2	1.46	2.415	3.360	0.222
	$k_{-1} \times 10^{-3} (min^{-1})$	9.104	9.293	10.440	10.464	1.155
	$(t_{1/2})_{ass.} (hr)$	0.400	0.360	0.330	0.300	2.600
	$(t_{1/2})_{diss.} (hr)$	1.26	1.240	1.100	1.100	10.000
BII	$k_a \times 10^9 (M^{-1})$	4.96	5.480	7.040	6.690	9.380
	$k_d \times 10^{-9} (M)$	0.201	0.182	0.142	0.149	0.106
	$k_{+1} \times 10^7 (M^{-1}.min^{-1})$	0.888	1.020	1.420	1.789	2.050
	$k_{-1} \times 10^{-3} (min^{-1})$	1.79	1.861	2.017	2.674	2.185
	$(t_{1/2})_{ass.} (hr)$	1.43	1.200	1.160	1.00	3.300
	$(t_{1/2})_{diss.} (hr)$	6.45	6.200	5.720	4.32	5.280
MI	$k_a \times 10^9 (M^{-1})$	0.294	0.592	2.792	7.590	0.229
	$k_d \times 10^{-9} (M)$	3.401	1.689	0.358	0.131	4.366
	$k_{+1} \times 10^7 (M^{-1}.min^{-1})$	0.632	0.804	1.325	1.977	0.120
	$k_{-1} \times 10^{-3} (min^{-1})$	21.496	13.581	4.745	2.605	5.240
	$(t_{1/2})_{ass.} (hr)$	2.700	0.93	0.800	0.500	2.800
	$(t_{1/2})_{diss.} (hr)$	0.53	0.85	2.420	4.430	2.200
MII	$k_a \times 10^9 (M^{-1})$	8.81	13.8	34.000	65.100	12.500
	$k_d \times 10^{-9} (M)$	0.113	0.072	0.029	0.015	0.080
	$k_{+1} \times 10^7 (M^{-1}.min^{-1})$	0.906	1.053	1.479	1.890	0.120
	$k_{-1} \times 10^{-3} (min^{-1})$	1.028	0.763	0.435	0.290	0.096
	$(t_{1/2})_{ass.} (hr)$	2.00	1.830	1.800	0.600	6.700
	$(t_{1/2})_{diss.} (hr)$	11.23	15.130	26.550	39.820	120.310

BI: Purified receptor No. 1 from benign tumors.

BII: Purified receptor No. 2 from benign tumors.

MI: Purified receptor No. 1 from malignant tumors.

MII: Purified receptor No. 2 from malignant tumors.

3.7.1.3. Estimation of Hill coefficients (n) of purified nuclear testosterone receptors

The Hill equation is an appropriate tool for binding analysis only when cooperativity is very strong or non–existent [192].

Figure (3–34) shows the Hill plots of ^{125}I-testosterone binding to its purified receptors in human benign and malignant prostatic tumors at 37°C.

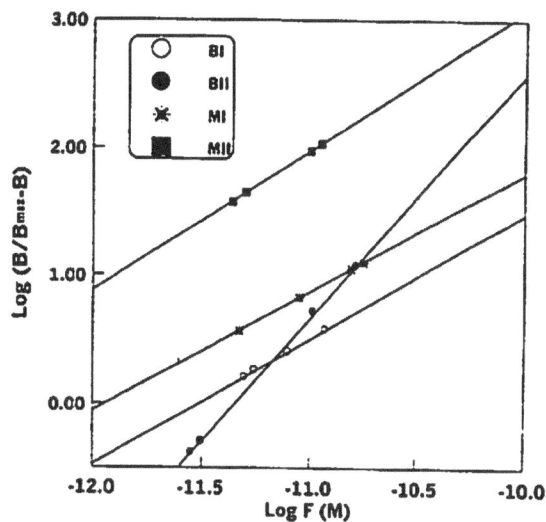

Figure (3-34): Hill plot of purified testosterone receptors at 37°C. All details are described in section (2.8.3).

Our results underlined that testosterone binding with its BI, MI and MII-purified receptors did not exhibit positive cooperativity during the binding reaction and the (n) values were 1.0, 0.916 and 1.09 respectively while the Hill analysis for BII-purified receptor confirms that there was a strong positive cooperativity (n ≅ 1.91) during the binding reaction and thus allosteric conformational changes occurred in the BII-purified testosterone receptor molecule upon binding with testosterone.

These results are in consistent with those reported previously by many investigators who underlined that androgen receptor from both calf uterine cytosol and human prostate tumor cell line (LNCaP) comprises three active domains: one for ligand binding, one for interaction with nuclear acceptor sites and a third domain which modulates nuclear interaction [174].

Other investigators showed that the mechanism of cooperative attachment of steroid hormone to its receptor is in dispute but two basic models have been proposed; the symmetrical, allosteric effector hypothesis of Monod and the induced fit, sequential hypothesis of Koshland [134].

Although Walent and Gorski (1990) presented a cooperative receptor model. According to this model, steroid (s) binds to a receptor and forms a nonactivated monomeric (SR) complex. The monomeric complex forms an activated (SR) dimer only after undergoing a cooperative dimerization reaction that is dependent on the concentration of (SR) monomeric complexes. Cooperative dimerization is therefore required for activation of (SR) complexes in this model[192].

3.7.2. The thermodynamics of the association of testosterone with its purified nuclear receptors

3.7.2.1. Thermodynamic parameters of standard state

Figure (3–35) represents the dependence of the affinity constant for the binding of ^{125}I-testosterone to its purified receptors in prostatic tumor homogenate on the temperature (Van't Hoff plot). From the results shown in Table (3-15), it was found that ΔH^o values of MI and MII were higher than that of BI and BII-purified receptors, so more energy is needed in case of malignant receptors for the reaction binding to occur. Also the negative value of ΔG^o was greater in purified receptor type-II than that of type-I in benign and malignant tumors, this may be attributed to the more reaction spontaneity and to the more stability of testosterone–receptor (II) complex than that of testosterone–receptor (I) complex. Table (3-15) also showed that ΔH^o and ΔS^o values for the binding of testosterone with its MI and also MII purified receptors were higher than with those of BI and BII purified receptors, this means that the short range interactions played an important role in stabilizing the malignant receptors complexes and the complexes formed possessed a less ordered structure than the testosterone and its malignant receptors compared with those of benign receptors.

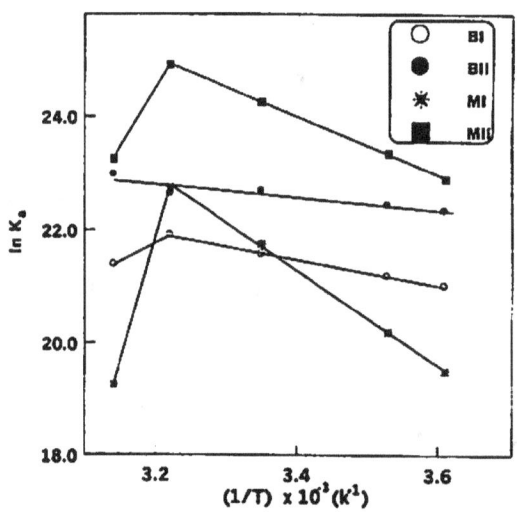

Figure (3–35): Van't Hoff plot for the ^{125}I-testosterone binding to its purified nuclear receptors. All details are described in section (2.8.4).

Table (3-15): Thermodynamic parameters at standard state of testosterone binding to its purified receptors in benign and malignant prostatic tumors. All details are described in section (2.8.4).

Purified receptor	Thermodynamic parameter	Temperature (°C)				
		4	10	25	37	45
BI	$\Delta H°$(kJ/mole)	+19.796	+19.796	+19.796	+19.796	+19.796
	$\Delta G°$(kJ/mole)	-48.365	-49.824	-53.424	-56.42	-56.52
	$\Delta S°$ (J/mole.K)	+246.068	+246.007	+245.704	+245.858	+239.987
BII	$\Delta H°$(kJ/mole)	+11.877	+11.877	+11.877	+11.877	+11.877
	$\Delta G°$(kJ/mole)	-51.416	-52.765	-56.181	-58.315	-60.711
	$\Delta S°$ (J/mole.K)	+228.494	+228.417	+228.382	+226.426	+228.264
MI	$\Delta H°$(kJ/mole)	+70.672	+70.672	+70.672	+70.672	+70.672
	$\Delta G°$(kJ/mole)	-44.910	-47.530	-53.889	-58.637	-50.896
	$\Delta S°$ (J/mole.K)	+417.263	+417.675	+417.990	+417.126	+382.290
MII	$\Delta H°$(kJ/mole)	+43.379	+43.379	+43.379	+43.379	+43.379
	$\Delta G°$(kJ/mole)	-52.740	-54.942	-60.084	-64.179	-61.472
	$\Delta S°$ (J/mole.K)	+347.0	+347.424	+347.191	+346.961	+329.720

3.7.2.2. Thermodynamic parameters of Transition State

Figure (3–36) shows the dependence of the association rate constant for the binding of ^{125}I-testosterone to its purified receptors on temperature (Arrhenius plot).

The results in Table (3-16) illustrate the effect of temperature on the thermodynamic parameters of the association of testosterone with its different nuclear purified receptors. These results also revealed that the values of E_a and ΔH^* for the binding of testosterone with its BI and MI–purified receptors was greater than those with BII and MII purified receptors, thus the reaction of testosterone with its BII and MII–receptors was easy to occur, so [^{125}I-testosterone-receptor type (II)]* formation required energy smaller to that required for [^{125}I-testosterone-receptor type (I)]* formation. This may be attributed to the structural differences between testosterone receptor and nuclear matrix. Also it was found that hydrophobic interactions play an important role in stabilizing the activated testosterone receptors complexes rather than that of nuclear matrix activated complex.

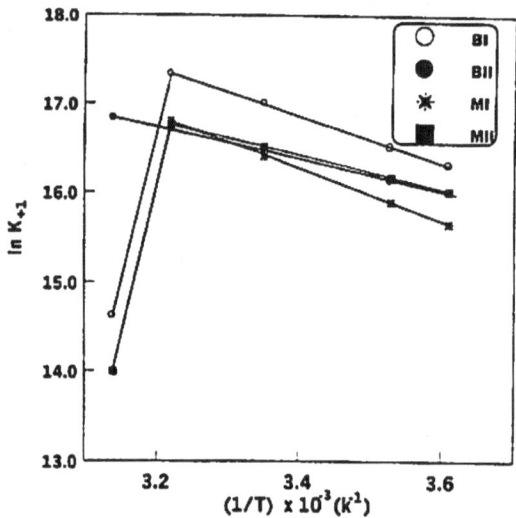

Figure (3–36): Arrhenius plot for the ^{125}I-testosterone binding to its purified nuclear receptors. All details are described in section (2.8.4).

Table (3-16): Thermodynamic parameters at transition state of testosterone binding to its purified receptors in benign and malignant prostatic tumors. All details are described in section (2.8.4).

Purified receptor	Thermodynamic parameter	Temperature (°C)				
		4	10	25	37	45
BI	E_a (kJ/mole)	+22.171	+22.171	+22.171	+22.171	+22.171
	ΔH^* (kJ/mole)	+19.868	+19.818	+19.693	+19.593	+19.527
	ΔG^* (kJ/mole)	+30.134	+30.367	+30.866	+31.360	+39.420
	ΔS^* (J/mole.K)	-37.061	-37.275	-37.493	-37.958	-62.556
BII	E_a (kJ/mole)	+15.441	+15.441	+15.441	+15.441	+15.441
	ΔH^* (kJ/mole)	+13.138	+13.088	+12.963	+12.863	+12.797
	ΔG^* (kJ/mole)	+30.825	+31.221	+32.184	+32.984	+33.543
	ΔS^* (J/mole.K)	-63.852	-64.074	-64.500	-64.906	-65.239
MI	E_a (kJ/mole)	+24.389	+24.389	+24.389	+24.389	+24.389
	ΔH^* (kJ/mole)	+22.085	+22.036	+21.911	+21.811	+21.745
	ΔG^* (kJ/mole)	+31.608	+31.779	+32.352	+32.726	+41.050
	ΔS^* (J/mole.K)	-34.379	-34.427	-35.037	-35.209	-60.707
MII	E_a (kJ/mole)	+16.130	+16.130	+16.130	+16.130	+16.130
	ΔH^* (kJ/mole)	+13.826	+13.777	+13.652	+13.552	+13.486
	ΔG^* (kJ/mole)	+30.779	+31.143	+32.080	+32.844	+41.050
	ΔS^* (J/mole.K)	-61.202	-61.364	-61.839	-62.232	-86.679

Most of the activation energy is due to the enthalpy term (19.868 kJ/mole for BI–receptors at 4°C); the activation energy due to the entropy term is much less and negative (about -10.265 kJ/mole). The magnitudes of these data rule out the possibility of covalent or ionic binding between testosterone and the BI-purified receptor. Dipole-dipole interactions of hydrogen bonds are typically 12.552–25.104 kJ/mole; therefore, assuming a single hydrogen bond per ketone, the one ketone group on testosterone could contribute from 12.552–25.104 kJ/mole to the binding. Our data suggest that the lower value of hydrogen bonding energy may be more reasonable. The rest of the binding (which could contribute about 7.316 kJ/mole) would be due to the induced dipolar interactions of Van der Waals' forces.

These interactions are inversely dependent on distance of separation to the sixth power and at the Van der Waals' radius can contribute typically 4.184 kJ/mole for each carbon-hydrogen group involved. Thus, for the minimum required Van der Waals' interactions, at least, and probably more than 1.748 atoms or about 9.2% of the testosterone molecular surface must be in close proximity to the receptor.

The same theoretical calculations [162] were repeated to another receptor types and at different temperatures, these results were listed in Table (3-17).

Table (3-17): Temperature effect on the number of (C-H) groups involved in Van der Waals' interactions and the testosterone molecular surface percent be in close proximity to the receptor.

Temp. (°C)	BI-purified receptor	BII-purified receptor	MI-purified receptor	MII-purified receptor
4	1.748 (9.2%)	n.d.	2.27 (11.94%)	n.d.
37	1.682 (8.85%)	n.d.	2.21 (11.63%)	n.d.
45	n.d.	n.d.	n.d.	n.d.

n.d.: Not detected.

From the values obtained from Table (3-17), it was concluded that the Van der Waals' interactions between testosterone and its receptors differ significantly depending primarily on the receptor type and this may reflect the different interactions nature between the testosterone and its receptors (I) and (II). These interactions are relatively strong in receptors type (I) compared with those in receptors type (II). Also it was found that the elevation of temperature decreases the strength of these interactions.

The results of temperature coefficient (Q_{10}) mentioned in Table (3-18) revealed that the increase in the association rate of testosterone with its receptors type (I) was greater than that with receptors type (II) by raising the temperature 10°C.

Table (3-18): Temperature coefficients (Q_{10}) of the binding of ^{125}I-testosterone with its purified benign and malignant prostatic receptors. All details are described in section (2.8.4).

Temp. ranges (°C)	BI-purified receptor	BII-purified receptor	MI-purified receptor	MII-purified receptor
273-283	1.412	1.271	1.461	1.285
283-293	1.379	1.251	1.424	1.263
293-303	1.350	1.232	1.391	1.244
303-313	1.324	1.216	1.362	1.227
313-323	1.302	1.201	1.336	1.211

Comparison of the thermodynamic parameters at the standard state and transition state of crude and purified testosterone receptors reveal the following notes:

1) ΔH° values of the purified receptors are more than that of the homogenate.

2) ΔG° values for the reaction of the purified and homogenate are nearly the same.

3) ΔS° values for the binding of testosterone with its benign purified receptors and the homogenate were nearly the same, while in the case of malignant receptors the ΔS° values for the binding of the purified receptors were more than that of homogenate. This increase was mainly attributed to the increase in the value of ΔH° since ΔG° for both (crude and purified) interactions had nearly the same values.

4) ΔH^{*}, ΔG^{*}, ΔS^{*}, E_a and Q_{10} values of the binding of benign and malignant purified testosterone receptors were more than that of the homogenate.

Finally comparison of Van't Hoff and Arrhenius plots for the different purified testosterone receptors reveal that at 45°C BII-purified receptor was the more thermostable form than the others.

3.8. Spectroscopic studies on human testosterone receptors

3.8.1 The U.V. spectra of purified testosterone receptors in human benign and malignant prostatic tumors

Figure (3–37 A&B) illustrates the U.V. spectra of purified testosterone receptors at pH 7.2. The U.V. spectra show that the λ_{max} for the purified receptor BI consists of two peaks; at 196 nm and 256.4 nm, BII-purified receptor gives one peak at 195.5 nm, MI-purified receptor gives one peak at 194 nm and MII-purified receptor gives one peak at 193.1 nm. As a result each human testosterone receptor has a characteristic spectrum and can be identified by their peaks. 196, 195.5, 194 and 193.1 nm are assigned to tyrosine residues, while the vibrational structure as a small "wiggles" at 256.4 nm is assigned to phenylalanine [193,194]. Also it was found from the Figure (3–37 A&B) that tryptophan residues does not occur on the surface of benign receptors while it slightly occurs on the surface of malignant receptors at 295 nm [194]. It seems that in BII, MI and MII-purified receptors, tyrosines are located in a way that part of it, is on the surface of the receptor molecules and the other parts are buried, whereas in BI–purified receptor, all tyrosine residues seem to be on the surface, exposed to absorbance. On the other hand, phenylalanine residues of the BI-receptor molecule seem to be on the surface, these residues partially buried in BII–receptor molecule while in MI and MII–receptors, these residues may be completely buried.

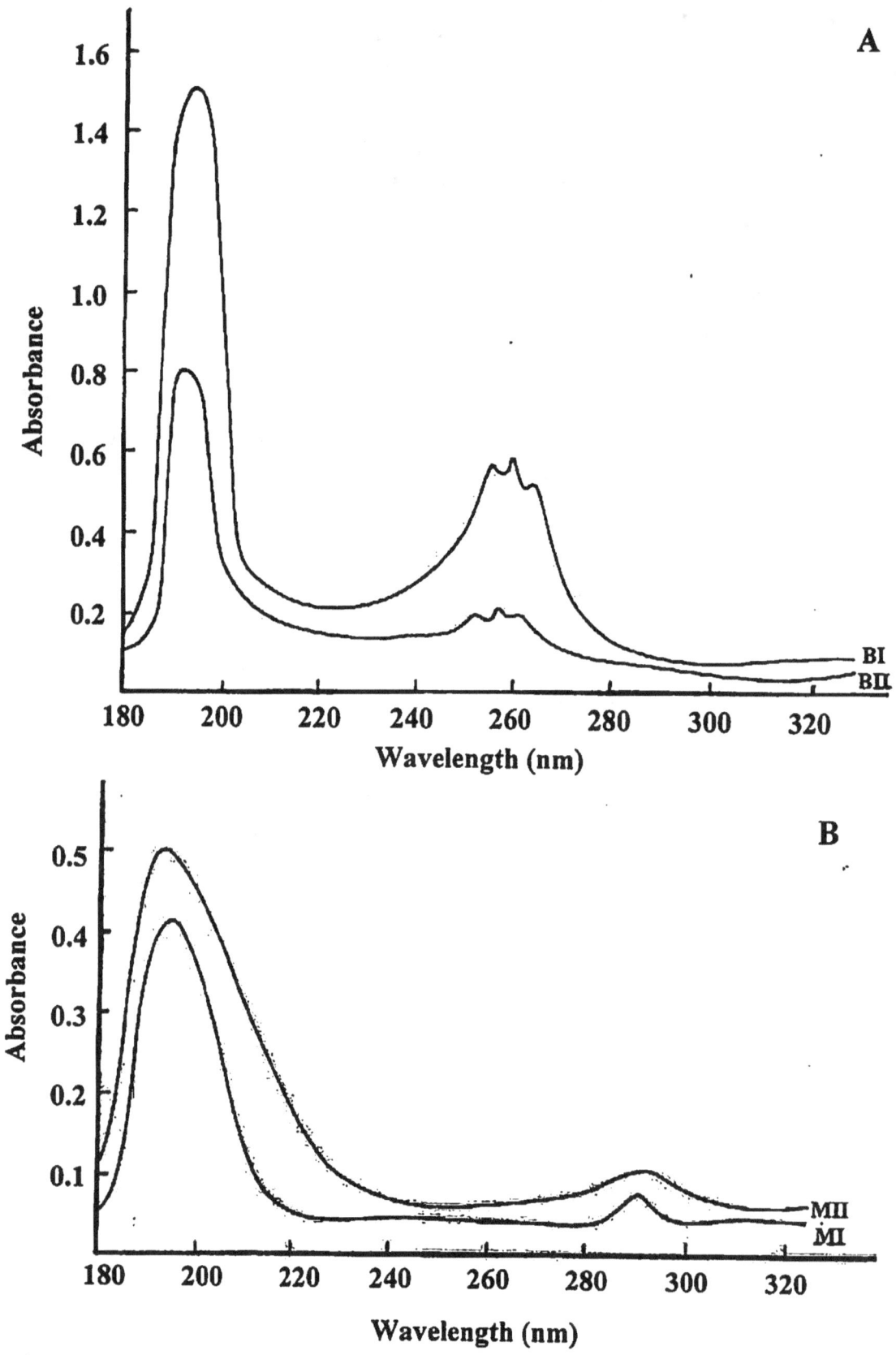

Figure (3–37): The U.V. spectra of purified nuclear testosterone, A) BI & BII receptors, B) MI & MII receptors. All details are described in section (2.9.1).

A trial to calculate the specific absorption coefficients (a_s) of human testosterone receptors revealed that $a_{s(196\ nm)}$ was found to be $8.85 \times 10^4\ cm^{-1}.g^{-1}.L$ and $a_{s(256.4\ nm)}$ was equal to $3.34 \times 10^4\ cm^{-1}.g^{-1}.L$ for BI–purified receptor, $a_{s(195.5\ nm)}$ was found to be $4.53 \times 10^4\ cm^{-1}.g^{-1}.L$ for BII–purified receptor, $2.61 \times 10^4\ cm^{-1}.g^{-1}.L$ was the $a_{s(194\ nm)}$ value for MI–purified receptor and $a_{s(193.1\ nm)}$ value for MII–purified receptor was found to be $3.06 \times 10^4\ cm^{-1}.g^{-1}.L$ according to the Lambert–Beer's law [110].

3.8.2. Factors affecting the absorption properties of testosterone receptors in human benign and malignant prostatic tumors

The absorption spectrum of a chromophore is primarily determined by the chemical structure of the molecule. However, a large number of environmental factors produce detectable changes in λ_{max} and ε. Environmental factors such as pH and polarity of the solvent provide the basis for the use of absorption spectroscopy in characterizing macromolecules [193].

3.8.2.1. pH effect

The pH of the solvent determines the ionization state of ionizable chromophores. Table (3-19) shows the λ_{max} values for human testosterone receptors at different pH (2-12). At an acidic pH 2. BI–purified receptor has four λ_{max} values at 206.1, 255.6 nm which were assigned to phenylalanine, 273 nm which was assigned to tyrosine and 293 nm which assigned to tryptophan residues.

In BII–purified receptor three λ_{max} were obtained at 209, 275 and 293.5 nm which were assigned to phenylalanine, tyrosine and tryptophan respectively. In MI–purified receptor, three λ_{max} were obtained, the first one at 221 nm, the second at 276 nm while the third at 294.0 nm, the first and the second peaks were assigned to tyrosine residues and the third one was assigned to tryptophan residues. In MII–purified receptor, one λ_{max} was obtained at 295 nm which was assigned to tryptophan.

At neutral pH 7.2, BI–purified receptor spectrum consists of two λ_{max}, the first at 196 and the second at 256.4 nm, these λ_{max} are assigned to tyrosine and phenylalanine respectively. In BII, MI and MII–purified receptors, there were one

λ_{max} at 195.5, 194 and 193.1 nm respectively which were assigned to tyrosine residues.

When the pH was increased from 8.2 to 9.2, there were no significant change in the λ_{max} obtained for each receptor type and the tyrosine is the only residue present in all cases but a further increase in pH value from 9.2 to 12 has shown an increase in the λ_{max} of tyrosine residues in all receptor types, this result is due to the dissociation of the phenolic OH of tyrosine ($pk_a = 10.07$) giving an ionized form of this amino acid which absorps at higher wavelength (red shift) [193].

In general, these results may be explained partly by the induction effects, so when the pH lowered from 12 to 6, the spectral maxima of tyrosine residues shift toward shorter wavelength (blue shift). This shift are due to slight increases in the energies of electronic transitions of the tyrosine aromatic ring, resulting from the formation of the electron–withdrawing ammonium group. Many researchers underlined that these inductive effects of vicinal charges are quite small to account for the changes occurring in protein spectra and the spectral shifts of proteins produced by changing pH must therefore be attributed mainly to rearrangements of secondary and tertiary structure, although the possibility of field effects, due to unusually close conjunction of charges to aromatic groups is not excluded [194].

Table (3-19): The effect of pH on the λ_{max} of testosterone receptors spectra. All details are described in section (2.9.2.1).

pH	BI-purified receptor λ_{max} (nm)	BII-purified receptor λ_{max} (nm)	MI-purified receptor λ_{max} (nm)	MII-purified receptor λ_{max} (nm)
2	206.1, 255.6, 273, 293	209, 275, 293.5	221, 276, 294	295
6	192.8	196.2	196.4	193.2
7.2	196, 256.4	195.5	194	193.1
8.2	193.2	193.1	192.8	192.4
9.2	193.5	193.8	192.8	195.4
12	295.5	295.1	295.2	295.3

3.8.2.2. Polarity effect on U.V. testosterone receptors spectra

1) The effect of 20% ethanol and dimethylsulfoxide (DMSO)

Table (3-20) shows the effect of 20% ethanol and dimethylsulfoxide at neutral pH on the testosterone receptors spectra. In 20% ethanol, it was found that one λ_{max} was obtained for each receptor, at 214, 213.8, 216.2 and 214.5 nm for BI, BII, MI and MII-purified receptors respectively which were assigned to tryptophan residues, while in the case of 20% DMSO, a newer λ_{max} was appeared for each purified receptor, these are 281.6, 282.6, 283 and 283.4 nm for BI, BII, MI and MII respectively which were assigned to tryptophan residues. The appearance of these new λ_{max} values indicates that the protein was defolded due to change in the secondary and tertiary structure of the protein that bring the tryptophan to expose to absorbance while phenylalanine and tyrosine residues were buried inside the receptor molecule, also it was found that testosterone receptors are highly sensitive to change in the polarity of the solvent.

2) The effect of 20% ethylene glycol

Table (3-20) and Figure (3–38 A&B) show the λ_{max} of human testosterone receptors BI and BII in 20% ethylene glycol at neutral pH. The data obtained previously in section (3.8.2.1) show that the λ_{max} of BI-purified receptor at neutral pH were 196 nm and 256.4 nm, the λ_{max} value of tyrosine was shifted towards longer wavelengths (red shift) in 20% ethylene glycol due to the hydrogen bonding of the OH groups of tyrosines with the solvent or with the π-electron system of the benzene ring where tyrosine was functioned as a hydrogen donor, while the λ_{max} value of phenylalanine was shifted towards shorter wavelengths in 20% ethylene glycol, this shift was attributed to $\pi \rightarrow \pi^*$ transitions [193,195]. These two shifts in λ_{max} were accompanied with an increase in the absorbency of phenylalanine and a decrease in the absorbency of tyrosine, these findings could be attributed to a change in the protein structure that bring the phenylalanine residues to the surface of the protein while tyrosine residues were partly embedded in a hydrophobic region of the protein molecule.

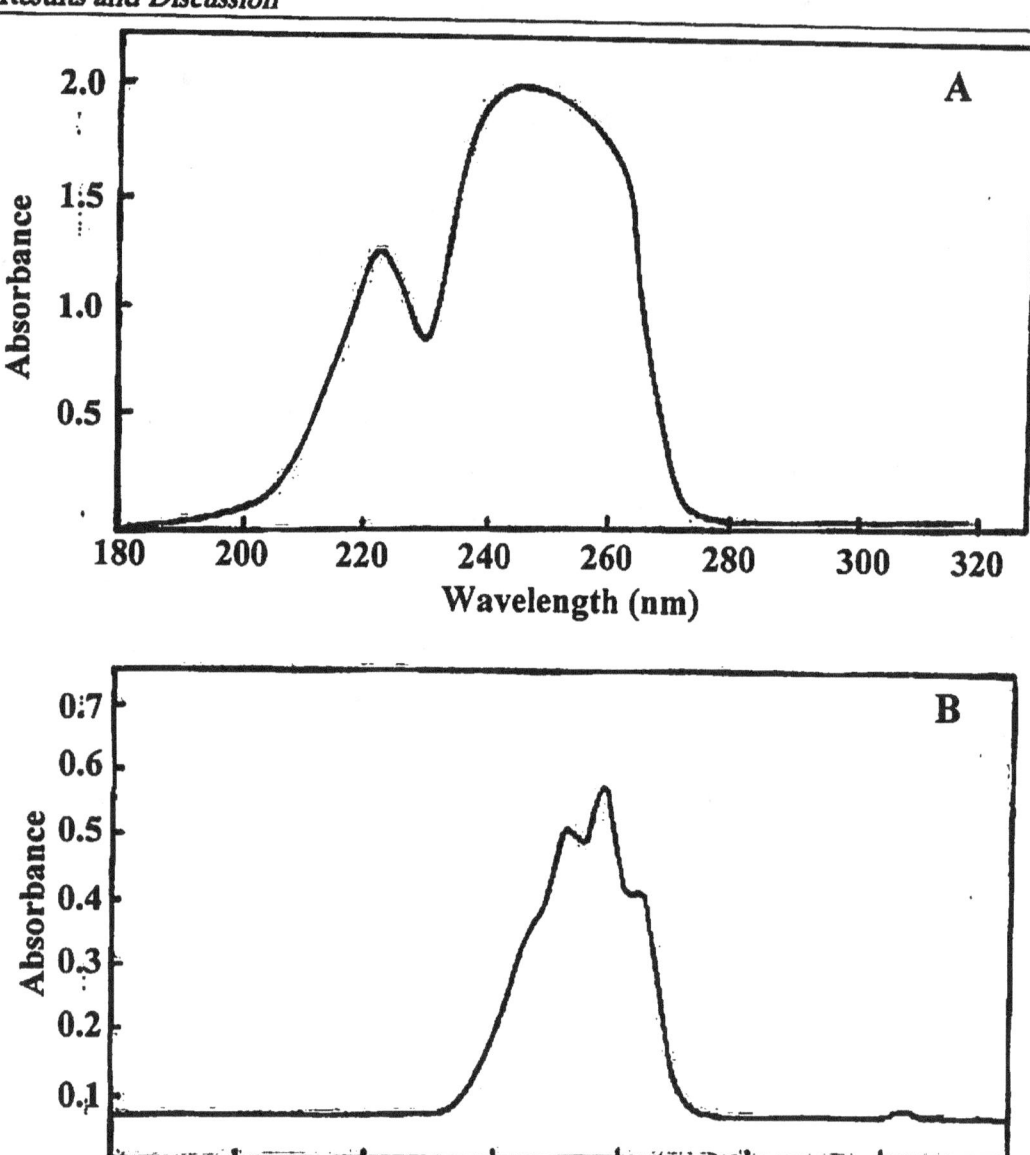

Figure (3–38): The effect of 20% ethylene glycol on, A) BI-purified receptor, B) BII-purified receptor. All details are described in section (2.9.2.2).

Table (3-20): The effect of 20% ethanol, ethylene glycol and dimethylsulfoxide on the λ_{max} of testosterone receptors spectra. All details are described in section (2.9.2.2).

Solvent	BI-purified receptor	BII-purified receptor	MI-purified receptor	MII-purified receptor
	λ_{max} (nm)	λ_{max} (nm)	λ_{max} (nm)	λ_{max} (nm)
20% ethanol	214	213.8	216.2	214.5
20% ethylene glycol	247.8, 222	257	-	-
20% DMSO	281.6	282.6	283	283.4

The changes in the protein structure for BII-receptor may bury tyrosine residues in the internal region of the protein and bring phenylalanine to the molecule surface. Also, it was found that malignant receptors were very high sensitive to ethylene glycol, this solvent can bury all absorbing amino acids inside the hydrophobic region of the protein molecule.

3) The effect of 20% urea

Table (3-21) shows the effect of urea on the testosterone receptors U.V. spectra at pH 7.2. Previous data in experiment (3.8.2.1) identified two peaks in BI-purified receptor spectrum, λ_{max1} at 196 nm and λ_{max2} at 256.4 nm at pH 7.2. These peaks were assigned to tyrosine and phenylalanine respectively. In the presence of 20% urea pH 7.2, these two amino acids were buried inside the receptor molecules and tryptophan residues were appeared on the surface. Similar effect was obtained on the MI-purified receptor molecules, since tyrosine residues were buried and tryptophan residues were appeared on the surface of molecule with a new absorption peak. The results indicate that urea affects the testosterone purified receptors BI and MI structurally, since many chromophores which were embedded in an interior region of the receptor molecule where they were inaccessible to the solvent came into contact with it due to the unfolding of the molecule, and hence, different spectra were obtained [195]. The λ_{max} of tyrosine residues in BII and MII-purified receptors were shifted towards longer wavelengths without affecting the structure of these receptors, the shift indicates that at 20% urea, the exposed tyrosines become solvated with urea (dipole–dipole interaction) [194,195].

Table (3-21): The effect of 20% urea on the λ_{max} values of testosterone receptors spectra at neutral pH. All details are described in section (2.9.2.2).

Purified receptor	λ_{max} (nm)
BI	293.21
BII	222.35
MI	295.28
MII	222.02

4) The effect of NaCl and CaCl₂

Table (3-22) shows the effect of NaCl and CaCl₂ on the U.V. spectra of testosterone receptors. The effect of these salts on increasing the binding extent of testosterone with its receptors in benign and malignant prostatic tumors ascertain us to study the effect of these salts on the testosterone receptors spectra. In BI-purified receptor, a blue shift was obtained in the λ_{max} of phenylalanine residues in the different salts used. This blue shift is due to the negative or positive charges of the salt anions and also cations which might interact directly with the π-electron system of the benzene ring of phenylalanine amino acids [195]. In all purified receptors, it was found that tyrosine residues were buried inside the interior region of the protein molecule and phenylalanine residues were appeared on the molecular surface of these receptors.

Table (3-22): The effect of NaCl and CaCl₂ on the λ_{max} values of testosterone receptors spectra. All details are described in section (2.9.2.2).

Solvent	BI-purified receptor	BII-purified receptor	MI-purified receptor	MII-purified receptor
	λ_{max} (nm)	λ_{max} (nm)	λ_{max} (nm)	λ_{max} (nm)
100 mM NaCl	205.4	204.8	205.0	205.4
25 mM CaCl₂	204.4	204.0	203.6	203.6

3.8.2.3. The effect of 10% cisplatin

The results in Table (3-23) show that cisplatin has no detectable effect on the λ_{max} positions of tyrosine residues in BI and BII-purified receptors, while phenylalanine residues on the surface of BI-receptor were embedded. In malignant purified receptors different effects were observed, these include the embedding of tyrosine residues inside the receptor molecule and the appearance of phenylalanine residues on the molecule surface, also a new absorption peak was appeared at 201.2 nm and 200 nm for MI and MII-purified receptors respectively, these λ_{max} values may be attributed to the receptor-drug complexes. Therefore, these results supported the results obtained previously in section (3.6) which reported that anticancer drugs might interact with malignant receptors but not with benign receptors.

Table (3-23): The effect of 10% cisplatin drug on the λ_{max} of testosterone receptors spectra. All details are described in section (2.9.3).

Purified receptor	λ_{max} (nm)
BI	195.65
BII	195.01
MI	244.2, 201.2
MII	246.3, 200

3.8.3. Spectrophotometric pH titration of purified testosterone receptors in human benign and malignant prostatic tumors

Spectrophotometric pH titration is the following of the change in absorbance of the chromophore with increasing pH [193]. Many studies of protein structure require the determination of pk values for proton dissociation from ionizable amino acid side chains, because these values give an indication of the location of the amino acid in the protein. This can often be done spectrophotometrically because dissociation often changes the spectrum of one of the chromophores, the observation of tyrosine dissociation was performed by measuring the absorption at 295 nm (λ_{max} for the ionized form of tyrosine), and the observation of histidine dissociation was carried out by measuring the absorption at 211 nm.

Figure (3–39 A&B) shows the pH titration curves of testosterone receptors for tyrosine and histidine respectively. (A) curves show that the pk_a values for tyrosine are 10.1, 11.5, 11.5 and 11.6 for BI, BII, MI and MII–purified receptors respectively, while the pk_a values for histidine in (B) curves were equal to 5.5, 7.48, 6.1 and 7.5 for BI, BII, MI and MII–purified receptors respectively. From the same figure, it was found that:

1) About 83.7, 91.8, 70 and 93.6% of tyrosine residues are located on the surface of the BI, BII, MI and MII–purified receptors molecule respectively.

2) About 16.3, 8.2, 30 and 6.4% of tyrosine residues are buried interior the folded structure of the BI, BII, MI and MII–purified receptors respectively.

3) About 91.8, 89.33, 99.2 and 90 % of histidine residues are located on the surface of the BI, BII, MI and MII-purified receptors molecule respectively.

4) About 8.2, 10.68, 0.8 and 10% of histidine residues are embedded in the interior region of the BI, BII, MI and MII-purified receptors molecule respectively.

5) In BI-purified receptor the tyrosine residues were largely present on the surface of the molecule and the internal tyrosines are in a strongly nonpolar environment, while the internal tyrosine residues in BII, MI and MII purified receptors were in a strongly polar environment (e.g. a tyrosine surrounded by carboxyl groups). On the other hand, the histidine residues are largely present on the molecular surface of BI and MI-receptors and the internal residues are in a nonpolar environment whereas the internal histidine residues of BII and MII-purified receptors are likely to be in a strongly polar environment.

6) Finally, the percent of external tyrosine residues in MII-purified receptor was greater than that of BII-purified receptor and the percent of internal tyrosine in MI-purified receptor was greater than that of BI-purified receptor, on the other hand the percent of internal histidine in BI-receptor was greater than that of MI-receptor and the percent in BII-receptor was greater than that of MII-receptor.

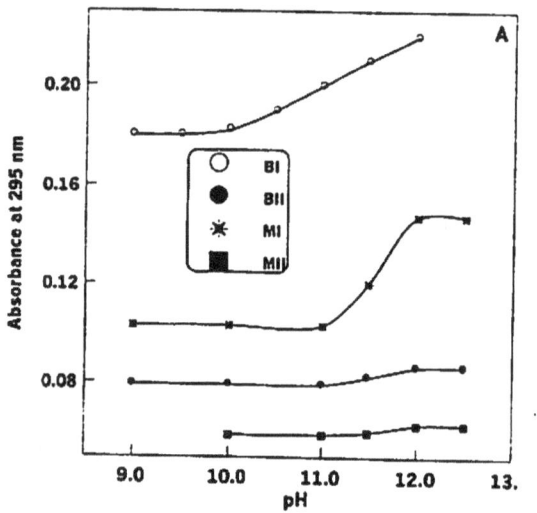 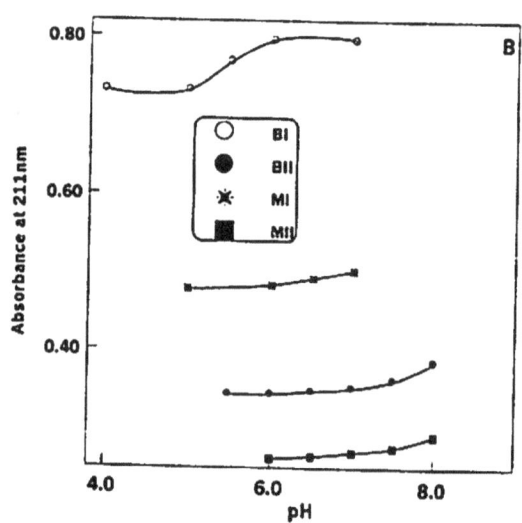

Figure (3–39): Spectrophotometric pH titration of purified nuclear testosterone receptors for, A) tyrosine residues, B) histidine residues. All details are described in section (2.9.4).

3.8.4. Determination of some aspects of the conformation of testosterone receptors by the solvent perturbation studies

The determination of whether an amino acid is internal or external by measuring the spectra of a protein in a polar and nonpolar solvents is called the solvent perturbation method. In fact, proteins are rarely studied in completely nonpolar solvents because most proteins are either insoluble or denatured in these solvents; therefore, mixtures of 80% water and 20% of reduced polarity solvent were used [193]. Solvents alter the peak positions and intensities by altering the energy and probability of electronic transitions and this alteration arises from a difference in the solvation energies of the ground state and the first excited singlet state [194].

Table (3-24) shows the λ_{max} and absorbance values in the absence and presence of different perturbants (20% ethanol, 20% ethylene glycol and 20% urea).

Table (3-24): Solvent perturbation on purified testosterone receptors. All other details are described in section (2.9.2).

Perturbing substance	BI-purified receptor		BII-purified receptor		MI-purified receptor		MII-purified receptor	
	λ_{max} (nm)	A	λ_{max} (nm)	A	λ_{max} (nm)	A	λ_{max} (nm)	A
Without	196 256.4	1.5 0.566	195.5	0.802	194	0.440	193.1	0.5
20% ethanol	214	0.081	213.8	0.072	216.2	0.080	218.5	0.076
20% ethylene glycol	247.8 222	1.998 1.285	257	0.574	-	-	-	-
20% urea	293.21	0.133	222.35	0.740	295.28	0.099	222.02	0.471

From the results listed in the Tables (3-20) and (3-24), it was found that several spectral changes were obtained in the presence of these perturbants, like the alteration of the λ_{max} positions and intensities of testosterone receptors spectra, and the appearance of new chromophores on the surface of the receptor molecule. These chromophores were embedded in an interior region of the protein in the absence of solvent.

From the solvent perturbation studies, the following remarks could be drawn:

1) About 83, 93.2, 70 and 93.3% of tyrosine residues are on the surface of BI, BII, MI and MII–receptor molecule respectively. So, about 25, 28, 21 and 28 tyrosine residues are on the surface of BI, BII, MI and MII–purified receptor molecule, while 19, 18, 21 and 19 histidine residues may be considered as external amino acids [185].

2) There are about 5 tryptophan residues in the benign receptor active site and 2 tryptophan residues in the malignant receptor active site. These results are in accordance with those obtained previously in section (3.2.2.12). Many investigators underlined that tryptophan residues present in the active site of androgen receptor and play an important role in the interaction with testosterone [134,152].

3.8.5. Observation of the helix-coil transition (denaturation) of purified nuclear testosterone receptors in human benign and malignant prostatic tumors

Because buried chromophore becomes exposed to the solvent during denaturation, by monitoring the absorbance of these chromophores, one can observe the helix–coil transition (denaturation) for proteins. For example, if a protein contains tryptophans, some of which are internal, the unfolding as a function of temperature could be detected by measuring the absorbance at 292 nm in a 20% ethylene glycol solution, also this could then be used to examine the effects of other agents such as NaCl concentration on the thermal stability. Figure (3–40 A, B, C&D) shows the thermal stability curves of purified testosterone receptors. The results obtained from these curves indicate that protein denaturation in 0.01 M–NaCl occurred at 50, 60, 40 and 50°C for BI, BII, MI and MII–purified receptors respectively, while in 0.1 M–NaCl the denaturation occurred at 60, 60, 40 and 60°C for BI, BII, MI and MII–purified receptors respectively, therefore, higher NaCl concentration causes more stabilization for the purified receptors. From the thermal stability curves, it was found that at 0.01 M–NaCl, BII–purified receptor was more thermostable than BI and MII–purified receptors and those were more stable than MI–purified receptor.

These results are in accordance with those reported previously by many investigators on nuclear androgen receptor of rat ventral prostate which indicated that these proteins are heat labile at temperatures above 50°C [138], also their heat-denaturation curve is similar to those obtained in our work.

Thermal stability analysis at 0.01 M-NaCl revealed that 6 tryptophan residues were embedded inside the internal region of BI and MII-purified receptors while 7 tryptophan residues were buried in an iterior region of the BII and MI-purified receptors.

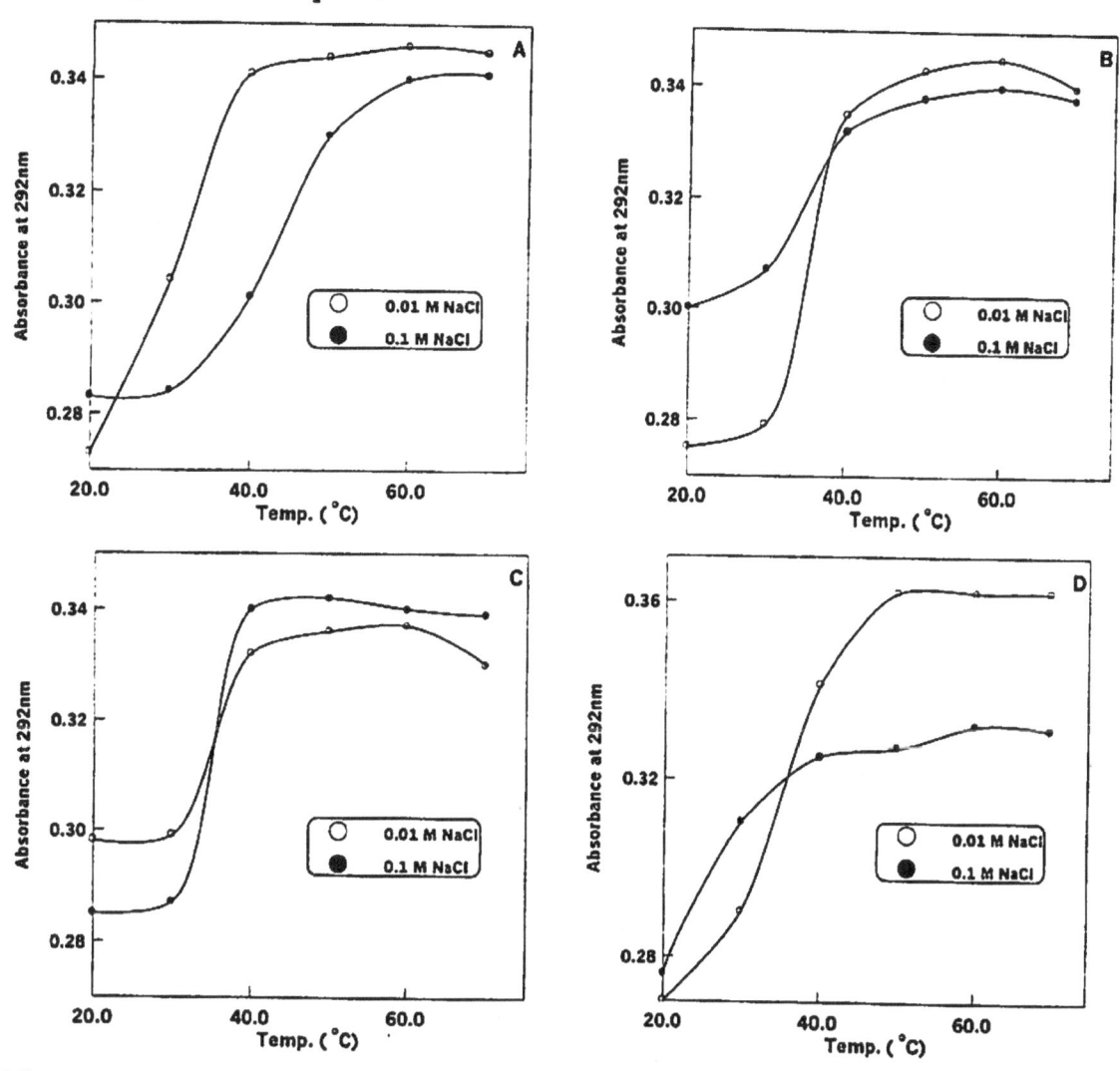

Figure (3–40): Helix-coil transition of purified nuclear testosterone, A) BI-receptor, B) BII-receptor, C) MI-receptor, D) MII-receptor with different NaCl concentrations. All details are described in section (2.9.5).

3.8.6. The U.V. spectra of ^{125}I-testosterone and of the different ^{125}I-testosterone-receptors complexes

The binding of ligand to the active site of a receptor frequently produces spectral changes in chromophores in or near the active site by affecting the polarity of the region or the accessibility to solvent this means that chromophores on the surface become inaccessible to the solvent by being buried in the region in which binding takes place or because a conformational change that buries or exposes a chromophore in another part of the molecule can accompany binding[193].

Table (3-25) shows the λ_{max} values of ^{125}I-testosterone and its complexes with purified receptors. Our results indicated that the binding of testosterone with its receptors abolished the λ_{max} values of free testosterone and also tyrosine residues were embedded in an interior region of the protein and appearance of phenylalanine residues on the molecule surface in all testosterone receptor types. Our results supported the previous steroid enveloping concept which suggests that testosterone is bound by its receptors from multiple sides (α, β and peripheral) and testosterone then is being "enveloped" in the hydrophobic cavity [138].

The absorbances at 213.6 and 267 nm obtained for testosterone may be attributed to the n$\rightarrow\sigma^*$, $\pi\rightarrow\pi^*$ and n$\rightarrow\pi^*$ electronic transitions respectively.

Table (3-25): The λ_{max} values of the U.V. spectra of ^{125}I-testosterone and its complexes with purified receptors. All details are described in section (2.9.6).

Purified receptor	λ_{max} (nm)
^{125}I-testosterone –R (BI)	204.6
^{125}I-testosterone –R (BII)	204.4
^{125}I-testosterone –R (MI)	205.6
^{125}I-testosterone –R (MII)	205
^{125}I-testosterone	213.6, 267

Conclusions

1. Serum copper to zinc and magnesium to calcium ratios may be introduced as biochemical markers in the discrimination between benign and malignant prostatic tumors patients.

2. The developed protocol for the assay of testosterone receptors is capable of analyzing these receptors and the procedure is suitable for the assessment of testosterone receptors in benign and malignant prostatic tumors.

3. A higher incidence of testosterone receptors was obtained in malignant than in benign prostatic tumors; therefore the malignant tumors were more testosterone dependent than those of benign tumors.

4. Two types of testosterone receptors are present in human benign and malignant prostatic tumors, the first one (I) was eluted with the void volume (V_o) while the second (II) was eluted with about 2.5 void volume (2.5 V_o).

5. The association of testosterone with its crude and purified benign and malignant prostatic tumors receptors were spontaneously occur ($\Delta G^o < 0$) and the binding reactions were entropically driven ($\Delta S^o > 0$).

6. BII-purified nuclear testosterone receptor was the more thermostable form at 45°C.

7. From the spectroscopic studies, it was suggested that the testosterone binding sites for all purified receptors are localized inside the receptor protein.

Future Work

According to the results obtained in this thesis, the following works are suggested for the future:

1. Evaluation of serum-TPS (tissue polypeptide specific antigen), salivary testosterone and other new tumor markers as possible markers in the early diagnosis and follow-up of patients with prostatic carcinoma.

2. Evaluation of the biological activity of testosterone receptors in human benign and malignant prostatic tumors.

3. Spectroscopical characterization of purified testosterone receptors by I.R., N.M.R., C.D., O.R.D., Fluorescence and x-ray diffraction analysis.

4. Immunohistochemical evaluation of the biological significance of proliferating cell nuclear antigen (PCNA) and nm 23 protein in human prostatic tumors tissues.

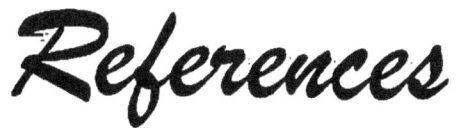

1. Kissane J.M.; **Anderson's Pathology**; 9th ed.; The CV Mosby Company; 1990; pp. 899-908.

2. Smith D.R.; **General Urology**; 10th ed.; Lange Medical Publications; 1981; p. 7.

3. Porth C.M.; **Pathophysiology: Concepts of Altered Health States**; 4th ed.; J.B. Lippincott Company–Philadelphia; 1994; pp. 87, 737-742.

4. Cockett A.T.K. and Koshiba K.; **Color Atlas of Urologic Surgery**; 1st ed.; Williams & Wilkins-USA; 1996; pp. 196-198, 204, 205.

5. Tanagho E.A. and McAninch J.W.; **Smith's General Urology**; 14th ed.; Prentice-Hall International Inc.; 1995; pp. 392, 393, 403-410, 424-427, 719-721.

6. Holland J.F., Bast R.C., Morton D.L., Kufe D.W. and Weichselbaum R.R.; **Cancer Medicine**; 4th ed.; Williams & Wilkins; 1997; pp. 2126-2137, 1133-1141.

7. McNeal J.E. and Fam A.; **The J. Urol.**; 1972; 107: 1008, 1022.

8. Mann C.V. and Russell R.C.G.; **Bailey and Love's Short Practice of Surgery**; 22nd ed.; Chapman and Hall Medical; 1995; p.970.

9. Brendler C.B., Berry S.J., Ewing L.L., McCullough A.R., Cochran R.C., Strandberg J.D., Zirkin B.R., Coffey D.S., Wheaton L.G., Hiler M.L., Bordy M.J., Niswender G.D., Scott W.W. and Walsh P.C.; **J. Clin. Invest.**; 1983; 71(5): 1114, 1122.

10. Meikle W., Stringham J.D. and Olsen D.C.; **J. Clin. Endo. Metab.**; 1978; 47(4): 909, 910.

11. Brendler C.B., Follansbee A.L. and Isaacs J.T.; **The J. Urol.**; 1985; 133: 495, 496.

12. Stege R. and Carlström K.; **J. Steroid Biochem. Molec. Biol.**; 1992; 42(3): 357, 361.

13. Hammond G.L.; **J. Endocrin.**; 1978; 78: 7, 8, 17.

14. Wilson J.D.; **The Amer. J. Med.**; 1980; 68 (Review): 745-749, 751-753.

15. Soxeland J; **Urology A Pocket Reference**; 2nd ed.; Thieme Flexi Book; 1989; pp. 254, 280.

16. Pusateri D.J., Roth W.T., Ross J.R. and Shultz T.D.; **The Am. J. Clin. Nut.**; 1990; 51(3): 371.

17. Biswas S; **Essentials of Pathology**; 1st ed.; New Central Book Agency (P) Ltd.; 1997; p. 666.

18. Javle P, Jenkins S.A., West C. and Parasons K.F.; **The J. Urol.**; 1996; 156: 1014-1019.

19. Burke S.R.; **Human Anatomy and Physiology for The Health Science**; 1980; p. 382.

20. McLough Lin. J. and Williams G.; **Br. J. Urol.**; 1990; 65(4): 313, 376.

21. Hold T; **Eur. Urol.**; 1994; 25(suppl. 1): 15.

22. Franks L.M.; **Cancer**; 1973; 32(5): 1092, 1141.

23. Laurence D.R., Bennett P.N and Brown M.J; **Clinical Pharmacology**; 8th ed.; Churchill Livingstone; 1997; p. 646.

24. Sanda M.G., Doehring C.B., Binkowitz B., Beaty T.H., Partin A.W., Hale E., Stoner E. and Walsh P.C.; **The J. Urol.**; 1997; 157: 876-879.

25. Lin M.F., Meng T.C., Rao P.S., Chang C., Schönthal A.H. and Lin. F.F.; **J. Biol. Chem.**; 1998; 273(10): 5939.

26. Chabner B.A. and Longo D.L.; **Cancer Chemotherapy and Biotherapy**; 2nd ed.; Lippincott-Raven Publishers–Philadelphia; 1996; pp. 64, 65, 71.

27. Juniewicz P.E., McCarthy M., Lemp B.M, Barbolt T.A., Shaw C., Hollenbaugh D.M, Winneker R.C., Reel J.R. and Batzold F.H.; **Endocrinology**; 1990; 126(5): 2625.

28. Dekker I.G., Tetu B., Janssen P.J and Van Der Kwast T.H.; **The J. Urol.**; 1996; 156: 1194-1197.

29. Ornstein D.K., Rao G.S., Smith D.S. and Andriole G.L.; **The J. Urol.**; 1997; 157: 880-884.

30. Steinber G.D., Carter B.S., Beaty T.L.; **J. Urol.**; 1990; 143: 131A.

31. Stege R.H., Tribukait B., Carlström K.A.M., Grande M and Pousette A.H.L.; **The Prostate**; 1999; 38: 183-188.

32. Cavalli F., Hansen H.H. and Kaye S.B.; **Text Book of Medical Oncology**; Martin Dunitz Ltd.; 1997; p. 185.

33. Klocker H., Culig Z., Hobisch A., Cato A.C.B. and Bartsch G.; **The Prostate**; 1994; 25: 266, 267, 269.

34. Crawford E.D.; **Cancer**; 1990; 66(5): 1035.

35. Carlström K., Stege R., Henriksson P., Grande M., Gunnarsson P. and Pousette A.; **The Prostate**; 1997; 31: 193-197.

36. Navratil H. and Pavone-Macaluso M.; **The J. Internat. Med. Res.**; 1990; 18(suppl.1): 3,26.

37. Kuil C.W. and Brinkmann A.O.; **Eur. Urol.**; 1996; 29(suppl. 2): 78-80.

38. Ekman P., Snochowski M., Dahlberg E., Bression D., Högberg B and Gustafsson J.; **J. Clin. Endo. Meta**; 1979; 49(2): 205.

39. Krieg M., Grobe L., Voigt K. D., Altenähr E. and Klosterhalfen H.; **Act. Endo**; 1978; 88: 397-407.

40. Carlström K. and Stege R.; **Br. J. Urol.**; 1997; 79: 427-431.

41. Syms A.J., Harper M.E. and Griffiths K.; **The Prostate**; 1985; 6: 145.

42. Williams R.H.; **Text Book of Endocrinology**; 5th ed.; W.B. Saunders Company; 1974; p. 1080.

43. Djiane J., Houndebine L. and Kelly P.A.; **Proc. Natl. Acad. Sci. (USA)**; 1981; 78: 7445.

44. Lawrence A.M and Landau R.L.; **Endocrinology**; 1965; 77(6): 1119.

45. Ghosh S.P., Chatterjee T.K. and Ghosh J.J.; **J. Reprod. Fert.**; 1983; 67: 235-238.

46. Burtis C.A. and Ashwood E.R.; **Tietz Text Book of Clinical Chemistry**; 3rd ed.; W.B. Saunders Company; 1999; pp. 723, 1602.

47. Van Nagell J.R., Donaldson E.S., Hanson M.B., Gay E.C. and Pavlik E.J.; **Cancer**; 1981; 48: 495.

48. Statland B.E.; **Diagn. Med.**; 1981; 4:2.

49. Tilton R.C., Balows A., Hohnadel D.C. and Reiss R. F.; **Clin. Lab. Med.**; Mosby-Year Book Inc.; 1992; pp. 285, 322.

50. Whitby L.G., Percy Robb I.W. and Smith A.F.; **Lecture Notes on Clinical Chemistry**; 3rd ed.; Blackwell Scientific Publications; 1984; pp. 381, 458.

51. Pandha H.S., Waxman J. and Sikora K.; **Br. J Hosp. Med.**; 1994; 51(6): 297.

52. Suresh M.R.; **Antican. Res.**; 1996; 16: 2273-2278.

53. Kaplan L.A. and Pesce A.J.; **Clinical Chemistry, Theory, Analysis and Correlation**; 2nd ed.; The C.V. Mosby Company; 1989; pp. 256, 610-612, 657, 730.

54. Varley H., Gowenlock A.H. and Bell M; **Practical Clinical Biochemistry**; 5th ed.; William Heinemann Medical Books Ltd.; 1980; pp. 917, 918.

55. Henry J.B.; **Clinical Diagnosis and Management By Laboratory Methods**; 19th ed.; W.B. Saunders Company; 1996; pp. 181, 278, 366.

56. Hasenson M., Lundh B., Stege R., Carlström K and Pousette Å; **The Prostate**; 1989; 14: 83-90.

57. Ruckle H.C. and Oesterling J.E.; **World J. Urol.**; 1993; 11(4): 227.

58. Haapiainen R.K., Permi E.J., Rannikko S.A.S., Voutilainen P.E.J., Liewendahl K., Stenman U.H. and Alfthan O.S.; **Br. J. Urol.**; 1990; 65(3): 264-267.

59. Stege R., Lundh B, Tribukait B., Pousette Å, Carlström K and Hasenson M.; **The J. Urol.**; 1990; 144: 299.

60. Stege R., Tribukait B., Lundh B, Carlström K, Pousette Å and Hasenson M.; **The J. Urol.**; 1992; 148: 833-837.

61. Polito M., Minardi D., Recchioni A., Giannulis I., De Sio G. and Muzzonigro G.; **Prostate**; 1997; 33(3): 208-216.

62. Patterson T, Weber T.H. and Ojala K.; **Clin. Chem.**; 1981; 27: 1147.

63. Effert P.J., McCoy R.H., Walther P.G and Lui E.T.; **J. Urol.**; 1993; 150: 257-261.

64. Fishman J.R., Gumerlock P.H., Meyers F.J. and Devere White R.W.; **J. Urol.;** 1994; 152: 202-207.

65. Green B. and Leake R.E.; **Steroid Hormones A Practical Approach**; IRL Press Limited; 1987; pp. 1, 64, 68, 72-78, 81, 82.

66. Litwack G.; **Biochemical Actions of Hormones**; New York and London Academic Press; 1972; p. 9.

67. Griffin J.E. and Ojeda S.R.; **Text Book of Endocrine Physiology**; Oxford University Press; 1988; pp. 43-46.

68. Jubiz W.; **Endocrinology A Logical Approach for Clinicians**; 2nd ed.; McGraw-Hill Book Company; 1985; p.5.

69. Lehninger A.L.; **Biochemistry**; Worth Publishers Inc. (USA); 1982; p. 724.

70. Berne R.M. and Levy M.N.; **Physiology**; 3rd ed.; Mosby Year Book; 1993; pp. 826,999, 1000.

71. Imura H. and Kuzuya H.; **Hormone Receptors and Receptor Diseases**; Excerpta Medica; 1983; p. 121.

72. Korolkovas A.; **Essentials of Medicinal Chemistry**; 2nd ed.; John Wiley and Sons (USA); 1988; pp. 1010, 1011.

73. Fletcher R.F.; **Lecture Notes of Endocrinology**; 2nd ed.; Blackwell Scientific Publications; 1978; p. 150.

74. Hiipakka R.A. and Liao S.; **Trends Endocrinol. Metab.;** 1998; 9(8): 319-321.

75. Liao S.; **J. Formos. Med. Assoc.;** 1994; 93(9): 744-747.

76. Murray R.K., Granner D.K., Mayes P.A. and Rodwell V.W.; **Harper's Biochemistry**; Twenty Second ed.; A Lange Medical Book; 1993; p. 519.

77. Mulder E., Vrij A.A. and Brinkmann A.O.; **Biochem. Biophysic. Res. Comm.;** 1983; 114(3): 1147.

78. Kaufman M., Pinsky L., Kubski A., Straisfeld C., Dobrenis K., Shiroky J., Chan T. and MacGibbon B.; **J. Clin, Endocrinol. Met.;** 1978; 47: 738.

79. Giannopoulo S.; **J. Biol Chem.;** 1973; 248 (3): 1004.

80. Ritzen E.M., Hagenäs L., Hansson V., French F.S. and Nayfeh S.N.; **J. Ster. Biochem.;** 1974; 5: 849.

81. De Boer W., Lindh M., Bolt J., Brinkmann A. and Mulder E.; **Endocri.**; 1986; 118(2): 851.

82. Giannopulos G.; **Biochem. Biophysica. Res. Comm.**; 1971; 44(4): 943.

83. Rawn J.D.; **Biochemistry**; International ed.; Neil Patterson Publishers (USA); 1989; p. 567.

84. **Coat-A-Count Total Testosterone RIA Kit**, DPC (USA).

85. Van Der Zon P; **The Lancet**; 1990; 336(8729): 1517.

86. Horton R., Hawks D. and Lobe R.; **J. Clin. Inves.**; 1982; 69: 1203.

87. Sánchezcarbayo M., Mauri M, Alfayate R., Miralles C. and Soria F.; **J. Clin. Chem.**; 1998; 44(8): 1744.

88. Morales A., Johnston B., Heaton J.P.W. and Lundie M.; **The J. Urol.**; 1997; 157: 849-854.

89. Husmann D.A., Wilson C.M., McPhaul M.J., Tilley W.D. and Wilson J.D.; **Endocrinol.**; 1990; 126(5): 3359, 3360.

90. Borkowski A., Body J.J. and Leclercq G.; **Eur. J. Can. Clin. Onco.**; 1988; 24(3): 509.

91. Smith D.F. and Toft D.O.; **Mol. Endocrinol.**; 1993; 7: 4-11.

92. Koivisto P., Kononen, J., Palmberg C., Tammela T., Hyytinen E., Isola J., Trapman J., Cleutjens K., Noordzij A., Visakorpi T. and Kallioniemi O.P.; **Canc. Res.**; 1997; 57: 314-319.

93. Shimazui T.; **Gan. TO. Kagaku. Ryoho.**; 1998; 25(6): 801-808.

94. Ris Stalpers C., Verleun Mooijman M.C., Trapman J. and Brinkmann A.O.; **Biochem. Biophysi. Res.**; 1993; 196 (1): 173-180.

95. Goy R.W. and Whalen R.E.; **Hormones and Behavior**; 1989; 23(1): 92,93.

96. Culig Z., Hobisch A., Hittmair A., Peterziel H., Cato A.C.B., Bartsch G. and Klocker H.; **The Prostate**; 1998; 35: 65.

97. Massa R. and Martini L.; **J. Steroid Biochem.**; 1974; 5(8): 941.

98. Honma Y. and Noumura T.; **J. Endocr.**; 1973; 59(3): 661,662.

99. Quarmby V.E., Beckman W.C. Jr, Cooke D.B., Lubahn D.B., Joseph D.R., Wilson E.M. and French F.S.; **Cancer Res.**; 1990; 50: 735-739.

100. Diamond D.A. and Barrack E.R.; **J. Urol.**; 1984; 132: 821-827.

101. Deutscher M.P.; **Methods in Enzymology**; Volume 182; Academic Press Inc.; 1990; pp. 31-38, 57, 197, 301-306.

102. **Clinical Assays, Gamma Coat Testosterone-^{125}I RIA Kit**; DiaSorin-USA.

103. Tietz N.W.; **Fundamentals of Clinical Chemistry**; 3rd ed.; W.B. Saunders Company–Philadelphia; 1987; pp. 520, 711, 712.

104. **Trace Elements in Human Nutrition and Health**; Publication from World Health Organization (WHO)-Geneva; 1996; pp. 76, 233.

105. Fauci A.S., Braun Wald E., Isselbacher K.J., Wilson J.D., Martin J.B., Kasper D.L., Hanser S.L. and Longo D.L.; **Harrison's Principles of Internal Medicine**; 14th ed.; Volume 1; McGraw Hill/Health Professions Division; 1998; p. 491.

106. Lowry O.H., Rosebrough N.J., Farr A.L. and Randall R.J.; **J. Biol. Chem.**; 1951; 193: 265-275.

107. Burton K.; **Biochem. J.**; 1956; 62: 315-323.

108. Liao S., Liang T., Fang S., Castañeda E. and Shao T.C.; **The J. Biol. Chem.**; 1973; 248(17): 6154-6162.

109. Scatchard G.; **Ann. Ny. Acad. Sci.**; 1949; 51: 660.

110. Segel I.H.; **Biochemical Calculations**; 2nd ed.; John Wiley and Sons; 1976; pp. 241, 278-281, 311, 326, 327, 373.

111. Dawes E.A.; **Quantitative Problems in Biochemistry**; Sixth ed.; Longman; 1980; pp. 112-118.

112. Scopes R.K.; **Protein Purification: Principles and Practice**; 2nd ed.; Springer-verlag; 1987; pp. 196-198.

113. **Gel Filtration Leaflet; Theory and Practice; Pharmacia-Fine Chemicals**; p. 46.

114. Bruchovsky N and Wilson J.D.; **The J. Biol Chem.**; 1968; 243(22): 5953.

115. Barrack E.R. and Coffey D.S.; **The J. Biol. Chem.**; 1980; 255(15): 7265.

116. Carlström K, Eriksson A., Stege R. and Rannevik G.; **Internat. J. Androl.**; 1990; 13: 67-73.

117. Johnson S.G., Joplin G.F. and Burrin J.M.; **Clin. Chem. Acta**; 1987; 163(3): 309-318.

118. Eriksson A. and Carlström K; **The Prostate**; 1988; 13: 249-256.

119. Habib F.K., Lee I.R., Stitch S.R. and Smith P.H.; **J. Endocri.**; 1976; 71: 99-107.

120. Delos S., Carsol J.L., Ghazarossian E., Raynaud J.P. and Martin P.M; **J. Ster. Biochem. Molec. Biol.**; 1995; 55(3-4): 375-383.

121. Hudson R.W.; **J. Ster. Biochem.**; 1987; 26(3): 349.

122. Walsh P.C., Hutchins G.M. and Ewing L.L.; **J. Clin. Inves.**; 1983; 72(5): 1772-1777.

123. Siiteri P.K. and Wilson J.D.; **J. Clin. Invest.**; 1970; 49: 1737.

124. Gloyna R.E., Siiteri P.K. and Wilson J.D.; **J. Clin. Inves.**; 1970; 49: 1746.

125. Bruchovsky N. and Lieskovsky G.; **J. Endocri.**; 1979; 80(2): 289.

126. Solomon N.W.; **Am. J. Clin. Nut.**; 1979; 32: 856.

127. Cavallo F., Gerber M., Marubini E.,; **Cancer**; 1991; 67: 738.

128. Cupta S.K., Shukla V.K., Vaidya M.P.; **J. Surg. Oncol.**; 1991; 46: 178.

129. Leake A., Chrisholm G.D., Busuttil A. and Habib F.K.; **Acta Endocr. Copenh.**; 1984; 105(2): 281-288.

130. Abdulla B., Dashti H., Hayat L.; **Metabolism of Minerals and Trace Elements in Human Disease**; Smith Gordon and Company Limited; 1989; p. 45.

131. Joan Reed M. and Stitch S.R.; **J. Endocri**; 1973; 58: 405-419.

132. Cohn D.V.,Talmage R.V. and Matthews J.L.; **Hormonal Control of Calcium Metabolism**; Excerpta Medica; 1981; pp. 79-85.

133. Haro L.S. and Talamantes F.G.; **Molec. Cellu. Endocri.**; 1985; 43: 199-204.

134. King R.J.B. and Mainwaring W.I.P.; **Steroid–Cell Interactions**; First ed.; The Butter Worths Company; 1974; pp. 10,11,18.

135. Kumar V.L., Wadhwa S.N., Kumar V. and Farooq A.; **J. Surg. Oncol.**; 1990; 44(2): 122-128.

136.Melander W. and Horvath C.; **Arch. Biochem. Biophysi.**; 1977; 183: 200-215.

137.Walsh M.P., Vallet B., Autric F.; **J. Biol. Chem.**; 1979; 254: 12136-12144.

138.Litwack G.; **Biochemical Actions of Hormones**; Volume IV; Academic Press; 1977; pp. 358, 364, 371, 372, 394.

139.Gong Y., Blok L.J., Perry J.E., Lindzey J.K. and Tindall D.J.; **Endocri.**; 1995; 163(5): 2172-2178.

140.Traish A.M., Muller E. and Wotiz H.H.; **The J. Biol. Chem.**; 1981; 256(23): 12028-12033.

141.Jensen E.V., Hurst D.J., DeSombre E.R. and Jungblut P.W.; **Science**; 1967; 158: 385-387.

142.Mainwaring W.I.P; **J. Endocri.**; 1969; 45: 531-541.

143.Haro L.S. and Talamantes F.G.; **Mol. Cell. Endocri.**; 1985; 41: 93.

144.Laurent T.C.; **Biochem. J.**; 1963; 89: 249.

145.Thompson T.C. and Chung L.W.K.; **Cancer Res.**; 1984; 44: 1019.

146.Nishigori H. and Toft D.; **Biochem.**; 1980; 19: 77-83.

147.Gaubert C.M., Tremblay R.R. and Dube J.Y.; **J. Ster. Biochem.**; 1980; 13: 931-937.

148.Nielsen C.J., Sando J.J., Vogel W.M. and Pratt W.B.; **J. Biol. Chem.**; 1977; 252: 7568-7578.

149.Miller L.K., Tuazon F.B., Mv E.N. and Sherman M.R.; **Endocrin.**; 1981; 108: 1309-1318.

150.Alexander N.H.; **Analy. Chem.**; 1958; 30: 1292-1294.

151.Patchornik A., Lawson W.B. and Witkop B.; **J. Am. Chem. Soc.**; 1958; 80: 4747, 4748.

152. Abelson D., Depatie C. and Craddock V; **Arch. Biochem & Biophys.**; 1960; 91: 71.

153.Geller J., Cantor T. and Albert J.; **J. Clin. End. Metab.**; 1975; 41(5): 854-862.

154. Snochowski M., Pousette A., Ekman P., Bression D., Andersson L., Högberg B. and Gustafsson J.; **J. Clin. Endocri. Metab.**; 1977; 45(5): 920.

155. Schröder F.H. and de Voogt H.J.; **Steroid Receptors: Metabolism and Prostatic Cancer;** Proceedings of a Workshop of the Society of Urologic Oncology and Endocrinology-Amsterdam; 1980; pp. 115, 116, 162, 220, 230, 259.

156. Sirett D.A.N. and Grant J.K.; **J. Endocrin.**; 1978; 77:101.

157. Ekman P., Snochowski M, Dahlberg E. and Gustafsson J.A.; **Eur. J. Cancer;** 1979; 15(2): 260.

158. Ekman P., Snochowski M, Zetterberg A., Högberg B. and Gustafsson J.A.; **Cancer;** 1979; 44(3): 1173-1174.

159. Benson R.C., Gorman P.A., O'Brien P.C., Holicky E.L. and Veneziale C.M.; **Cancer;** 1987; 59(9): 1604, 1605.

160. Brinkmann A.O., Bolt J., Van-Steenbr-Ugge G.J., Kuiper G.G., de-Boer W. and Mulder E.; **Prostate;** 1987; 10(2): 133-143.

161. Weiland G.A. and Molinoff P.B.; **Life Science;** 1981; 29: 314-315.

162. Seeley D.H., Wang W.Y. and Salhanick H.A.; **Biochem. Biophys. Acta;** 1980; 632: 538.

163. Lea O.A. and French F.S.; **Cancer Res.;** 1981; 41: 619.

164. Nemethy G. and Scheraga H.A.; **J. Phys. Chem.;** 1962; 66: 1773-1789.

165. Waelbroeck M., Van Obberghen E. and DeMeyts P.; **J. Biol. Chem.;** 1979; 254: 7736-7740.

166. Kauzmann W.; **Adv. Prot. Chem.;** 1959; 14: 1-63.

167. Ross P.D. and Subramanian S.; **Biochem.;** 1981; 20: 3096.

168. Blumenthal D.K. and Stull J.T.; **Biochem.;** 1982; 21: 2386-2391.

169. Laporte D.C., Wierman B.M. and Storm D.R.; **Biochem.;** 1980; 19: 3814.

170. Donnelly B.J., Lakey W.H. and Mcblain W.A.; **The J. Urol.;** 1984; 131(4): 806.

171. Gonor S.E., Lakey W.H. and Mcblain W.A.; **The J. Urol.;** 1984; 131(4): 1196.

172. Castagnetta L., Carruba G., Fecarotta E., Lo-Casto M., Cusimano R. and Pavone-Macaluso M.; **Urol. Res.;** 1992; 20(2): 127-132.

173. Mainwaring W.I.P. and Irving R.; **Biochem. J.;** 1973; 134: 113.

174. Mulder E., Van Loon D., DE Boer W., Schuurmans A.L.G., Bolt J., Voorhorst M.M., Kuiper G.G.J.M. and Brinkmann A.O.; **J. Ster. Biochem.;** 1989; 32(1B): 151-155.

175. Johnson M.P., Young C.Y.F., Rowley D.R. and Tindall D.J.; **Biochem.;** 1987; 26(11): 3147-3182.

176. Hansson V., Tveter K.J., Attramadal A. and Torgersen O.; **Act. Endocri.;** 1971; 68: 79-88.

177. Sullivan J.N. and Strott C.A.; **The J. Biol. Chem.;** 1973; 248(9): 3202-3208.

178. Unhjem O. and Tveter K.J.; **Act. Endocri.;** 1969; 60: 571-578.

179. Mainwaring W.I.P. and Milroy E.J.G.; **J. Endocr.;** 1973; 57(3): 371-384.

180. Unhjem O.; **Act. Endocri.;** 1970; 65(3): 517-524.

181. Unhjem O., Tveter K.J. and Aakvaag A.; **Act. Endocri.;** 1969; 62: 153-164.

182. Rosen V., Jung I, Baulieu E.E. and Robel P; **J. Clin. Endocr. Metab.;** 1975; 41(4): 761-770.

183. Fang S. and Liao S.; **The J. Biol. Chem.;** 1971; 246(1): 16-24.

184. Rennie P. and Bruchovsky N.; **The J. Biol. Chem.;** 1972; 247(5): 1546-1554.

185. Heyns W., Peeters B., Mous J., Rombauts W. and De Moor P.; **Eur. J. Biochem.;** 1978; 89(1): 181-186.

186. Steins P., Krieg M., Hollmann H.J. and Voigt K.D.; **Act. Endocri.;** 1974; 75: 773-784.

187. Shain S.A. and Boesel R.W.; **Invest. Urol.;** 1978; 16(3): 169-173.

188. Berkovitz G.D., Brown T.R. and Migeon C.J.; **Clin. Endocr. Metab.;** 1983; 12(1): 155-173.

189. Trachtenberg J and Walsh P.C.; **The J. Urol.;** 1982; 127(3): 466-470.

190. Benson R.C., Utz D.C., Holicky E. and Veneziale C.M.; **Cancer;** 1985; 55(2): 382-388.

191. Rowley D.R., Thompson S.A., Lubaroff D.M. and Heidger P.M.; **Prostate**; 1984; 5(1): 101-111.

192. Walent J.H. and Gorski J.; **Endocr.**; 1990; 126(5): 2383-2391.

193. Freifelder D.; **Physical Biochemistry**; 2nd ed.; 1982; pp. 500-503, 511-517.

194. Yanari S. and Bovey F.A.; **J. Biol. Chem.**; 1960; 235(10): 2818-2825.

195. Leach S.J. and Scheraga H.A.; **J. Biol. Chem.**; 1960; 235(10): 2827, 2828.